SELF-
CARE
FOR INTROVERTS

17 SOOTHING RITUALS FOR
PEACE IN A HECTIC WORLD

BARRIE DAVENPORT

Self-Care for Introverts: 17 Soothing Rituals for Peace in a Hectic World

Publishing services provided by:

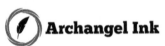 **Archangel Ink**

ISBN: 978-1-7320350-3-4

Disclaimer

Your Free Gift

As a way of saying thank you for your purchase, I'm offering a free companion website that is exclusive to readers of *Self-Care for Introverts*.

With the companion website, you'll have access to a collection of printable guides, checklists, questions, and other bonuses. Copy and paste the link below into your browser to get free instant access.

selfcareintroverts.com

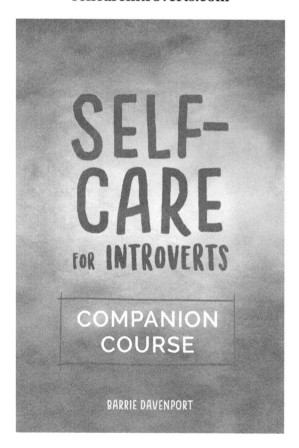

Contents

About Barrie Davenport

Barrie Davenport is a certified personal coach, thought leader, author, and creator of several online courses on mindfulness, relationships, self-confidence, life passion, habit creation, and self-publishing She is the founder of the top-ranked personal development site, Live Bold and Bloom.com. Her work as a coach, blogger, and author is focused on offering people practical strategies for living happier, more successful, and more mindful lives. She utilizes time-tested, evidence-based, action-oriented principles and methods to create real and measurable results for self-improvement.

You can learn more about Barrie on her Amazon author page at barriedavenport.com/author.

Introduction

In the summer of 2012, I attended a conference in Portland, Oregon, with the auspicious name, "The World Domination Summit." The purpose of the summit was focused on a central question as posed by the event founder (author, blogger, speaker, and world traveler Chris Guillebeau): "How can we live a remarkable life in a conventional world?"

At the time, hundreds (and now thousands) of people attended the event to inspire one another and learn ways to be remarkable and unconventional, especially as online experts and thought leaders. Eager to learn more about building my new business as an online entrepreneur and self-improvement blogger, I signed up and traveled across the country to join this "movement" of people who wanted to make an impact.

Given the name of the summit and the demeanor of most of the attendees I saw around me, I was woefully out of my natural element as an introvert (behind my computer, writing). Dominating the world is not high on my list of desired life goals. Even so, I knew it was valuable to absorb new ideas and hobnob with others in the industry, so I pushed myself out of my comfort zone.

One of the featured speakers was someone I hadn't heard of before, but I was intrigued and eager to hear her speak because of the topic and her newly released book related to it. The speaker was Susan Cain, author of the book *Quiet: The Power of Introverts in a World That Can't Stop Talking.* Since her talk that day, Cain's book has sold millions of copies, has been on the *New York Times* bestseller list for several years, and was named the number one best book of the year by *Fast Company* magazine.

Susan Cain has become the de facto spokesperson for introverts, having one of the highest viewed TED talks* (on the topic of introversion) and lecturing regularly at top-notch organizations and universities, helping introverts and extroverts understand how they have an equally valuable and important role to play in our work, relationships, and culture.

Who knew the subject of introversion would be so fascinating to so many? Certainly most introverts wouldn't have guessed it, having spent years fretting:

"Why do I feel so different?"

"Can't I just stay home and curl up with a book?"

"Don't these people have something more interesting to talk about?"

At one point or another, most introverts have viewed themselves as outlanders, the less-desirable cousins to their gregarious, outgoing, and extroverted peers.

As I conducted research on the 2012 World Domination Summit (the one I attended) to confirm dates and speakers to include in this book, I discovered an online marketing page for the event. The summit was clearly geared toward more extroverted world dominators, but there was an effort to make introverts feel more comfortable.

We have bands coming in from faraway lands. Our Bollywood DJ will return for an encore performance. The world's finest hammocks will be hung throughout the lobbies. We'll have yoga in the park, a 200-person photo walk through the Pearl District, a mass book signing with 20 authors, and an attempt to set some sort of Guinness world record.

It will be big... but not TOO big. A mobile site will allow attendees to connect with each other based on shared interests and location, ensuring that plenty of small-group gatherings can take place. A "highly-sensitive person" lounge will welcome the introverts among us.
—Save the Date! Announcing the 2012 World Domination Summit

Perhaps the lounge for introverts was a nod to Susan Cain and her participation in the summit, but I never knew it existed until today, as I'm writing this introduction. The Bollywood DJ never announced where to find it, and even if it was announced, I doubt there would have been a rush of sensitive people wanting to lounge.

How could anyone feel comfortable lounging quietly to take care of themselves and have any hope of being remarkable or unconventional? Even the introverts at the event knew they had to feign enthusiasm and energy and be brightly sociable to add any value or seem relevant. Little did I know, as I was faking my way to world domination, that my own assumptions about introverts were about to be turned upside down.

Back in the main theater, I sat on the edge of my seat, riveted by the information Susan Cain was sharing about her research on introverts. I'd only recently confirmed I was an introvert myself, after years of wondering why I always wanted to leave parties early and why I got so agitated in shopping malls and at concerts.

Before my online career, I'd worked as a public relations professional for more than twenty years. I knew what it felt like to pretend to be extroverted in an industry that favored outgoing, charismatic people. I'd experienced the tremendous energy toll it took to put myself out there in front of a group, to compete for an editor's attention and interest, or to serve as the smiling spokesperson for an organization.

What I loved about my former public relations career wasn't hanging out with designers, reporters, or celebrities. It wasn't talking on camera or making speeches. It wasn't organizing and attending big events. Yes, I did plenty of those things, but they made me weary and unsettled.

What I really loved was researching and writing press releases and speeches, collaborating with my peers and clients in small meetings, and brainstorming new ways to promote a product or make some extroverted personality shine in the spotlight.

During the early years of my public relations career, I couldn't identify why exactly I felt so uncomfortable with the "public" aspect of public relations. I just pushed through, knowing what was expected of me and observing how my extroverted peers were scrambling and competing for the spotlight. So I followed along.

It seems a lot of introverts do this—they fake extroversion. They fake it because society rewards extroversion and even suggests that introverts are not quite right in the head. They are shy, awkward, or lacking self-confidence. In our culture (particularly Western culture), being a friendly, congenial, ebullient conversationalist and an outspoken leader are venerated qualities. Introverts are often overlooked, ignored, and even mocked for their more reserved preferences.

Susan Cain has changed the world's perceptions about introverts, bringing the quiet, taciturn, and more contemplative among us out of the shadows and into, if not the spotlight, the warm glow of lamplight, where we can thrive, knowing we have as much to contribute as our extroverted friends.

Susan Cain's book has served as a beacon of inspiration and validation for the millions of introverts who, according to Cain's research, make up a third to a half of the world's population. If you are an introvert, you are in the company of some powerful, but quiet, world dominators—Abraham Lincoln, Bill Gates, Eleanor Roosevelt, Albert Einstein, Mahatma Gandhi, Rosa Parks, Warren Buffett, Steven Spielberg, and Barack Obama, to name a few.

Understanding how you operate in the world and validating your own worthiness as an introvert is extremely valuable for your self-esteem, relationships, and personal motivation. But that awareness doesn't change the fact that you are still operating in a culture that favors the extrovert ideal. It is like being left-handed (as I am) in a right-handed world. You know there's nothing wrong with you, but, nonetheless, most everything is geared for right-handers.

How can introverts truly thrive in this culture of outspoken world dominators? How can we take care of ourselves to ensure we perform optimally? How can we protect our more sensitive, reserved, and quiet natures, so we don't burn out or lose ourselves in the noise and activity around us?

Self-Care for the Self-Aware Introvert

Living in an extroverted world means we can't expect those around us to naturally intuit or respond to our needs. We must be mindful and proactive ourselves. Despite our newly minted standing as normal folk, it is up to us to manage our lives in a way that nurtures our strengths and tends to our unique needs.

That is the purpose of this book—to give you guidance on the proper self-care and maintenance of your quiet powers of world domination.

In every aspect of your life, from your personal relationships to your career, to your social life, your introverted nature will affect your experiences, for both good and ill. With some self-awareness and planning, you can find the proper balance and calibration of your time, experiences, and interactions to help you enjoy life to the fullest, have satisfying relationships, and maintain your physical and mental health.

You might currently find yourself in relationships and environments that are well-suited to your introverted preferences, and you feel quite comfortable and confident. But sooner or later, you'll be called on to step into a highly stimulating environment or engage with people who are extroverted. These situations shouldn't be feared or avoided altogether because they can enhance your life, expand your horizons, and enliven your mood—to a point.

Knowing how to bring yourself back to center, to take care of your emotional and physical needs, manage your social life, and set relationship boundaries allows you dip in and out of the extroverted world without crumbling or exhausting yourself.

Throughout this book, we will dive into these areas of your life and outline how you, as an introvert, can take action to protect, pamper, and prepare yourself to flourish in an extroverted world. Before we dive in, however, let's review just a little about what makes you an introvert, how you differ from extroverts, and why you are so valuable to the world.

A Little about Introverts

If you call yourself an introvert, you likely know something about the qualities and preferences that are part of an introvert's nature. You might have read books and articles and taken assessments on the subject. Introverts tend to be self-reflective and curious, so learning more about yourself is a natural instinct.

However, you might be late to the game in recognizing yourself as an introvert. Closet introverts often go undetected in social circles and in the hallways of business, and some introverts even fool themselves—sometimes for decades. They don't wake up to their true natures until something big happens, like a job loss, an empty nest, or even a mid-life crisis.

Perhaps you've struggled for years to fit in with the extroverts around you and don't understand what's "wrong" with you. You're just realizing that what's wrong isn't wrong at all, and you want to learn more about your unique qualities and how you can live more authentically.

Or maybe you're not an introvert but rather an ambivert or an extrovert who has a special introvert in your life. You want to understand what motivates this important person and how you can best support him or her. If so, bravo for you! Introverts need the care, understanding, and support of their loved ones to really shine and thrive.

Although this book is focused on *self-care* for introverts, it's beneficial for anyone reading to have a little refresher on personality type and what makes an introvert an introvert—whether you have a PhD in introvertology or you are still trying to connect the dots.

Let's start with the fact that introversion is a *perfectly normal* personality trait held by a quarter to a half (depending on the studies you read) of the population. Being introverted doesn't mean you are shy or have social anxiety.

There's nothing wrong with you, weird about you, or less valuable than your extroverted peers. You possess gifts and skills that are powerful and essential to your own success and even to the success of our culture. More on that in a moment.

If you've wondered where the identifications of introversion and extroversion gained a foothold, turn your attention to the early twentieth century and a Swiss psychologist named Carl Jung. The traits of introversion and extroversion are foundational to the theories of personality type and were first popularized by Jung in his 1924 book *Psychological Types*.

The well-known Myers-Briggs Type Indicator* was developed to make the theory of Jung's psychological types more understandable and useful in people's lives. Virtually every other model of personality typing, such as the Big Five personality traits, includes the traits of introversion and extroversion.

Of course, the traits themselves have been around since the dawn of time. Evolutionary psychologists suggest that the history of these types reaches back to some of the earliest members of the animal kingdom, from fruit flies to pumpkinseed sunfish to rhesus monkeys. Both introverts and extroverts make appearances in the Bible and in the writings of Greek and Roman physicians.

But it wasn't until centuries later that we began to look at ourselves and wonder if our personalities were up to snuff. Says Susan Cain in her book, *Quiet*, "The word *personality* didn't exist in English until the eighteenth century, and the idea of 'having a good personality' was not widespread until the twentieth" (page 21).

The "Extrovert Ideal," as Cain calls it, was de rigueur by the early 1900s, as the United States made the transition from a primarily rural to an urban society. With more people moving to cities and living among strangers, it became necessary to make quick and favorable impressions on other people.

America was also becoming more industrialized and entrepreneurial, requiring those who wanted to succeed in the new economy to "sell" ideas and products to other people.

In this brave new world, shimmering with possibilities, those with charisma, sociability, gregariousness, and leadership abilities were viewed as the clear champions. Those without these skills were doomed to sit on the sidelines writing poetry and eating beans from a tin can. Or so it was believed.

Fortunately, Carl Jung's work on personality type opened a window of understanding about the natural differences between the "doers" and the "thinkers" of the world. According to Jung's type theory, extroversion and introversion explain different attitudes people use to direct their energy—outward or inward.

The two traits are viewed as a continuum, whereby individuals can possess qualities of both, with one being more dominant than the other. Even extremes of both traits do not always act according to their type. For example, you might notice as an introvert that you enjoy socializing to a point, or that you don't mind the spotlight if it's in small doses.

In general, introverts are focused more on internal thoughts, ideas, memories, imagery, feelings and moods rather than seeking external stimulation. Unlike extroverts, who are energized by social interactions, introverts *expend* energy in social situations and can feel drained after spending too much time in a large group of people. They often need to "recharge" by spending a period of time alone.

In addition, introverts tend to . . .

- prefer one-on-one conversations to group activities;
- prefer to express themselves in writing;
- enjoy solitude;
- care less about wealth, fame, and status than their peers;
- be good listeners;
- avoid risk-taking;
- enjoy engaging deeply in work with few interruptions;
- prefer small-scale interactions, with only a few close friends or family members;
- prefer not to show or discuss their work with others until it's finished; and
- think before they speak.

—Excerpted from Susan Cain's "Quiet Revolution Personality Test"*

If you aren't sure where you fall on the introvert/extrovert continuum, consider taking the Myers-Briggs assessment or another personality assessment that measures these two traits. You can easily find them online.

Understanding how introverted you are can help you determine the ways you most need to protect and care for yourself, where you can stretch yourself, and how you can manage your life, so you thrive rather than feel depleted and overwhelmed.

It also inspires you to better appreciate your introverted nature and educate those around you that being an introvert is not only perfectly acceptable but also advantageous in many ways—in your personal and professional lives.

The Uncommon Powers of Introverts

As an introvert, you have impressive strengths that are nurtured by your more quiet and thoughtful nature. Because you don't have to rely on others for your energy and inspiration, you can tap a wellspring of deeply considered ideas and insights.

Your calm and steady mind picks up on subtleties that others wouldn't notice, and this sensitivity makes you incredibly valuable as an employee, friend, and love partner.

"Introverts focus on depth versus breadth," says Jennifer Kahnweiler,* author of the book, *Quiet Influence: The Introvert's Guide to Making a Difference.* As a result, you listen more than you talk—an attractive quality in itself, but one that is uniquely natural for introverts.

Your active listening skills help you make strong personal connections and enjoy deep and satisfying relationships with a smaller number of people. Active listening and keen observation contribute to another introvert skill—writing. Introverts are excellent writers, easily conveying what they've heard, observed, and pondered in the written word.

Introverts have more gray matter in the prefrontal cortex, the area of the brain that processes abstract thought and reflection. As *New York Times* bestselling author John Green muses, "Writing is something you do alone. It's a profession for introverts who want to tell you a story but don't want to make eye contact while doing it."*

Introverts are also careful in their choices of friends and romantic partners. They don't arbitrarily pick people to be in their lives, and their connections are deep and intimate. Introverts are intensely loyal to those they care about. They are often the people their friends turn to in difficult times because of their calm, measured approach toward problem-solving.

Skilled at planning, prioritizing, and focusing, introverts are some of the most reliable, creative, and disciplined people on the planet, able to follow through and get things done while others are still talking or having meetings.

Because of your ability to concentrate and process information, you often prepare better than others, being more informed and making creative connections that others don't see. Feeling good about yourself now? Wait, there's more!

In the workplace, a new view is emerging that's no longer associated with the shy, reclusive loner who is too meek to stand up for himself or reach for the golden ring. According to new research, it appears introverts possess qualities and strengths that are powerful and world-changing at work.

Some of the most successful, wealthiest entrepreneurs—like Warren Buffett, Bill Gates, and Larry Page—are introverts and built their businesses using the introvert's most highly valued skills: deep thinking, introspection, active listening, and quiet confidence.

As the world becomes more technologically oriented, globally connected, and entrepreneurial, introverts will experience a new level of respect and influence.

As science journalist Winifred Gallagher reminds, "The glory of the disposition that stops to consider stimuli rather than rushing to engage with them is its long association with intellectual and artistic achievement. Neither E=mc2 nor Paradise Lost was dashed off by a party animal."*

Of course, the best scenario is one in which the party animals and the quiet thinkers of the world respect the strengths and talents each bring to the table and work side by side toward common goals and achievements. The more freedom that introverts have to contemplate solutions and ideas, the more opportunities will be available to extroverts to implement them.

This is all good news for introverts who are gaining new respect and prestige for what they offer both personally and professionally. But what does all of this new respect mean for our happiness and well-being? Does it require us to be more available to others, to overextend ourselves in the wake of finding our footing in society?

I've often wondered how Susan Cain (who is an introvert) handled the success of her blockbuster book, having to go on book tours, make speeches, and endure dozens of interviews. Where we once had to suffer being stigmatized in silence, we now might suffer less but we might be missing some of the silence.

How to Use This Book

Perhaps now more than ever it's important for introverts to pay attention to our well-being and manage our lives in a way that energizes rather than depletes us. Now that we are noticed for our contributions, insights, and creativity, we might need to protect ourselves from the very thing we longed for—recognition and acceptance from others.

What's far more important for introverts, however, is *self*-awareness and *self*-acceptance, which allows us to step back, assess our unique needs from a position of strength, and take the necessary actions that protect us from feeling overwhelmed and sapped of our vitality.

What happens when you don't take these actions and overextend yourself? You probably know from experience. Maybe you recognize these signs.

- You feel agitated and foggy, unable to communicate or create properly.
- Everything irritates you, even people and activities you normally enjoy.
- You are extra self-critical and can feel guilty for no reason.
- You ruminate so much, your brain aches.
- You have no tolerance for small talk.

- You crave time alone to the point that you risk being rude to others.

- You're physically and emotionally drained.

- You feel anxious and/or depressed.

Practicing self-care is a way of showing respect for yourself and embracing your introverted nature by tending to the unique needs that are part of it. This book is divided into two sections related to these needs: physical self-care and mental and emotional self-care. Within each section, you will find detailed strategies for the unique challenges and requirements of introverts.

All the self-care actions outlined might not apply to you or your circumstances, and you certainly wouldn't have time to employ them all anyway—unless you want to spend every waking hour with self-care. Simply reading about these activities will make you more aware of your own needs. But reading alone isn't enough.

As you read, highlight actions you want to practice and incorporate in your daily life. If you'd like, keep a journal to write down the self-care actions that resonate with you, so you can revisit them later and determine when and how you want to add them to your daily routine.

At the end of the book, I've included a list of additional resources, sectioned by chapter, that might be helpful as you continue to explore your introverted nature and how to take care of it.

SECTION 1

PHYSICAL SELF-CARE

"To keep the body in good health is a duty . . . otherwise we shall not be able to keep our mind strong and clear."

—Buddha

As an introvert, your physical self-care is more important than you might realize. You have certain susceptibilities that can affect your health and overall fitness if you don't pay attention. But with self-awareness and some simple behavior changes, you can be as hearty as your extroverted friends who have a slight edge when it comes to their health.

So why do extroverts have a health advantage? It appears that extroverts might have stronger immune systems than introverts. A 2014 joint study* conducted by the University of Nottingham and the University of California, Los Angeles, suggests that people who were more extroverted had an increased expression of the genes that regulate the body's pro-inflammatory response.

Those who scored high in "conscientiousness" on the Big Five personality test (the more introverted participants) had reduced expression of these genes. This makes introverts more susceptible to infectious diseases, and chronic illnesses that affect introverts can often take a more serious course.

It seems extroverts have immune systems that can deal more effectively with infection, perhaps because they are more social and therefore exposed to more germs than introverts.

Introverts Must Prioritize Exercise

Introverts also might be less likely than extroverts to join a gym or participate in group fitness classes. Group fitness holds the potential for socializing and making small talk, not to mention suffering with loud music and large open spaces—anathemas to most introverts.

In a 2011 study* on personality type and body weight, the lead researcher, Angelina R. Sutin, PhD, noted that "lifestyle and exercise interventions that are done in a group setting may be more effective for extroverts than for introverts."

Because you are "in your head" so often, you might resist or neglect exercise altogether, preferring to sit still and read a book, write, or perform some other quiet and solitary activity. But as much as you might resist it, exercise is an introvert's best friend, helping you out of your head and into your body for a short period of time.

Managing stress is one of the main reasons introverts must prioritize exercise. It's no secret that stress and anxiety have a negative impact on anyone's physical well-being. It can cause headaches, gastrointestinal problems, cardiovascular issues, inflammation, and even problems with the reproductive systems of both men and women.

Introverts tend to experience a higher degree of stress (and depression and anxiety) about certain situations, like being with unfamiliar people, speaking in front of groups, and other stimulating scenarios. As an introvert, you need to work harder to manage stress and anxiety to protect your health.

Exercise not only reduces stress, it makes you feel better, sleep better, maintain your ideal weight, live longer, stay healthier, and helps reduce the negative self-talk that being in your head so much can foster. You simply can't not do it.

Exercise is also a mindfulness activity that forces you to stay present and focused on the performance of your body and the physical goal you are trying to achieve. We'll talk more about the importance of mindfulness in Section 2.

For now, just know that daily exercise is an essential part of your self-care as an introvert. I'll detail some specific fitness programs that are good for introverts later in this section.

Too Much Isolation Is a Risk Factor

Although introverts are energized by spending time alone, too much isolation is a risk factor for health problems and a shorter lifespan. Also, when you spend time alone, you might be prone to brooding and rumination, which can interrupt sleep or make it hard to fall asleep.

In fact, introverts have a propensity for sleep disorders, and a lack of sleep can lead to chronic fatigue and even depression. That's why it's critical to your health that you find the right balance of solitude and socializing.

If you're a more "extroverted introvert," this won't be as difficult for you. But if you are an introvert through and through, you'll need to make a concerted effort to spend time with your close circle of friends and family on a more regular basis.

It might be uncomfortable, but it's necessary for your long-term health. The positive part of social stimulation for you is that socializing exhausts you, increasing your need for sleep, which can elude you when you are isolated for long periods.

Dealing with Your White Coat Syndrome

As an introvert, you might have a hard time making doctor's appointments and getting checkups because the interaction with the doctor or the medical setting makes you anxious. Your overactive mind might make you ruminate about "worst case" scenarios, wondering if that annoying symptom might be a dire disease.

You can't stand sitting in crowded waiting rooms and being poked and prodded by even the kindest nurses and doctors. You might even resist speaking up with questions for your doctor, resulting a in lower standard of healthcare.

In general, introverts tend to feel drained more quickly, especially after a day at work or socializing with others. You sense all stimuli more intensely than your extroverted counterparts. As a result, it is particularly important for you to pay attention to your body's needs, protect yourself, and rejuvenate to increase energy. You want to find the balance between too much and too little stim- ulation, what psychologists call "the optimal stimulation level."

Although it might sound like introverts have a dire prognosis when it comes to their health and fitness, the health conditions outlined here do not manifest in the lives of every introvert.

If you practice the self-care techniques outlined in the subsequent chapters, you can manage the stressors that make you susceptible to exhaustion, illness, sleep deprivation, and too much isolation. And you can take actions that ensure you are keeping your body and your overall health in peak form.

In Section 1, we'll go through these eight physical self-care strategies.

1) Find the right workout.

2) Practice mindful fitness.

3) Create a well-care plan.

4) Get plenty of sleep.

5) Pay attention to your body.

6) The introvert diet.

7) Body and skin care rituals.

8) Creating your introvert retreat.

Let's get started!

Chapter 1
Find the Right Workout

"True enjoyment comes from activity of the mind and exercise of the body; the two are ever united."

—Wilhelm von Humboldt

It's clear that exercise is essential for your health and well-being, and as an introvert, you'd probably prefer to exercise from the comfort of your home or by taking a solitary run.

Exercising by yourself is better than not exercising at all, and for some introverts, solitary workouts are a necessity. But you can address two introvert challenges at once if you join a small group class or work with a personal trainer.

Remember, too much isolation isn't good for you, and joining a small class or training with a partner gives you a relatively manageable way to socialize without having to put yourself out there too much.

- Find a local gym that offers classes and ask about the classes that are the least attended or that are intentionally small.
- Or ask one or two friends to join you in paying for small group personal training sessions.

I've found a small personal training gym near my home that never has more than five or six people working out at any one time. I work with a trainer and have some moments of enjoyable conversation with him in between sets. And I can interact with some of the other clients whom I've gotten to know over time. It's the perfect setup for me, as I work from home and spend a lot of time by myself.

Being accountable to friends or to a trainer can ensure you follow through with your exercise program, at least on the days you attend a class or go to the gym. Even if you can't find a small class, you can supplement your solitary workout with a larger class once a week.

Try to scope out a trainer or class instructor who fits with your introverted nature. The gregarious instructor who is more of a cheerleader or Tony Robbins' style motivator might drain you before you even get winded with exercise. You'll do better with a more low-key, down-to-business vibe that doesn't make you feel like the wallflower at a fraternity party.

You also might prefer a class that has more of an individual component to it, like a spin class or Pilates, where you have your individual equipment, and you aren't required to do partner work and chat it up with others.

If taking any kind of group classes feels draining, set aside time on the days you participate in classes to regroup and find your center again. Rather than heading right back to work or to another social gathering, take some time by yourself to meditate, read a book, or listen to some music.

Create the buffer and transition you need to engage in your next activity. Or plan your class workout at a time when you know you can go home and recharge.

Chapter 2
Practice Mindful Fitness

"Movement is a medicine for creating change in a person's physical, emotional, and mental states."

—Carol Welch

There are a variety of fitness activities that cultivate mind-body integration and support an overall practice of mindfulness, which is so valuable for introverts. We will cover mindfulness in the next section, but for now, it's important to know that mindfulness helps you stay present and engaged in what you are doing so your overactive mind doesn't distract and agitate you.

It helps reduce stress and provides a restorative buffer against your tendency to experience anxiety and depression. When you practice a fitness routine that involves mindfulness, you are once again gaining multiple benefits by taking care of your physical well-being and training your mind to stay focused and attentive to the task at hand.

You can certainly apply mindfulness to any exercise you perform by keeping yourself focused on your breathing and being present with each physical action you perform. But this is often easier said than done. Your introverted brain has a wandering mind of its own, especially with exercise that doesn't require much concentration.

You can facilitate more focus and presence by adopting exercise routines that have a mindfulness component built into them. Below are several mindful fitness activities you might consider, which can be practiced in a class or by yourself following an instructor on a video.

You might need to combine some of these with an aerobic activity if you need more of a cardio workout, but these programs can help you build strength, flexibility, coordination, and balance.

Yoga

The word yoga is a Sanskrit word, derived from the word *yuj*, which means to yoke, as you'd yoke a team of oxen. This definition is often interpreted as meaning union, and yoga is said to unite the mind, body, and spirit. Yoga is about creating balance in the body through stretching and flexibility, and awareness in the mind through concentration on poses.

Yoga is especially good for introverts because:

- It enhances concentration as you focus on performing various poses.
- It increases flexibility and muscle tone, which improve your confidence.
- It enhances mindfulness, making you less prone to rumination.
- It encourages physical and mental balance to reduce stress.
- It develops proper body alignment, which makes you appear more confident.

- It promotes a sense of calm and peace necessary for mental health.

- It increases lung capacity for better breathing and improved focus and concentration.

There are many styles of yoga practices, all with varying exercises, philosophies, and desired outcomes. Hatha yoga is the most widely practiced form of yoga and is one of the six original branches of yoga. It uses movement and breath together to produce a "flow" of postures that lead from one to the next.

For the purpose of mindful fitness, yoga is a program of physical poses (asanas) designed to purify the body and provide physical strength and stamina. It works with the energy in the body, through pranayama or energy control.

Prana also refers to breath, and yoga teaches us how to use breath control to still the mind and attain higher states of awareness. A beginning yoga class might include the following asanas.

Initial Relaxation

At the beginning of the class, the students lie on their backs in a relaxed pose while breathing deeply. The teacher will guide students through a relaxation exercise where students alternately tense and release various parts of the body. The combination of deep breathing and tension/release helps calm the mind and relieve tension in the body.

Sun Salutations

The sun salutation is a sequence of twelve yoga positions performed at the start of every yoga class as a warm-up. Dozens of muscles are stretched and toned in this yoga exercise, as the sequence is performed several times.

Shoulder Stand

The shoulder stand is an inverted pose that increases the blood supply to the brain, by lifting your legs perpendicular to the floor and resting your weight on your shoulders, neck, and head and supporting your back with your hands. It exerts a gentle pressure on the neck region, which helps regulate the functions of the thyroid gland (which governs metabolism).

Fish Pose

With this pose, you stay flat on your back and bring your feet together. With your arms straight by your sides, you tuck your hands underneath your buttocks. Then you arch your spine and tilt your head so that your crown rests on the ground and hold the pose for thirty seconds. This yoga pose energizes the thyroid gland and enhances the flexibility of the upper back.

Forward Bend

With this yoga pose, you inhale and take the arms up over the head and lift and lengthen up through the fingers and crown of the head. You exhale and slowly lower the torso toward the legs. Reach the hands to the toes, feet, or ankles. This stretches the entire back of the body, increasing the flexibility of the lumbar spine and improving postural alignment. It also gives a nice massage to the abdominal organs.

Triangle Pose

The triangle is a standing yoga pose with a sideways-bending movement that simultaneously stretches, contracts, and relaxes all major back muscles, making the spine more elastic. It also provides a deep stretch for the hamstrings, groins, and hips.

Final Relaxation

Again, students lie on their backs and are guided through active relaxation (tensing and releasing muscles), deep breathing, and a visualization exercise to end the class.

In a typical class, the teacher might go through many more poses than just these, as there are hundreds of different yoga poses. Any of these poses can be practiced for a few minutes during the day as a brief mindfulness practice to refocus your attention on your body and to relax and calm you.

If you would like to take a beginning yoga class online, check out the DoYogaWithMe* site for a variety of tutorials. You can also try the 5 Minute Yoga, Daily Yoga, or Simply Yoga apps for your Android or iPhone.

Tai Chi

Tai chi began in China as a martial art, but as it developed, it took on the purpose of enhancing physical and mental health. It is a series of low-impact, weight-bearing, and aerobic movements that create internal balance and harmony and encourage the proper flow of qi, the energy force within the body.

There are a variety of styles of tai chi, but they all involve slow, circular, gentle movements, deep breathing and meditation—sometimes called "moving meditation."

As you perform the movements, you breathe deeply and naturally, focusing your attention on bodily sensations. Tai chi requires the practitioner to spend long periods of silent self-analysis (sound familiar, introverts?) with little stimulus, while using a slow rhythm, making it a perfect practice for introverts.

It is believed to improve the flow of energy in the body, leading to healthy living and providing a wide range of benefits, such as improved mood, more energy and stamina, and increased agility and flexibility. The practice of tai chi has a calming and meditative effect that reduces stress and anxiety.

Says tai chi master T. T. Liang in his book, *T'ai Chi Ch'uan for Health and Self-Defense: Philosophy and Practice,*

> *Of all the exercises, I should say that T'ai Chi is the best. It can ward off disease, banish worry and tension, bring improved physical health and prolong life. It is a good hobby for your whole life, the older you are, the better. It is suitable for everyone—the weak, the sick, the aged, children, the disabled and blind. It is also an economical exercise. As long as one has three square feet of space, one can*

take a trip to paradise and stay there to enjoy life for thirty minutes without spending a single cent (page 11).

A tai chi class can include the following elements.

Warm-Up

Easy motions to help loosen your joints and muscles and help you focus on your breath and body.

Instruction and Practice of Tai Chi Forms

Forms are sets of movements that might include a dozen or fewer movements. Long forms might include hundreds of movements. Focusing the mind solely on the movements helps produce a state of mental calm and clarity.

Breath Work

This consists of a few minutes of gentle breathing, sometimes combined with movement. The idea is to relax the mind while mobilizing the body's energy. It might be practiced standing, sitting, or lying down.

If you are interested in learning tai chi, visit Online Tai Chi Lessons* for a variety of classes you can take. Also check out the T'ai Chi For Life* app for iPhones and iPads, where each sequence is shown with clearly annotated diagrams and accompanied with a detailed text description.

Qigong

Qigong is a form of Taoist yoga, which is similar to tai chi, suggesting that the health of the mind and body is dependent on a clear, strong balance flow of qi or life force. The benefits of qigong extend to every physical system of the body, in addition to the mental, emotional, and spiritual aspects.

Qigong is an integration of physical postures, breathing techniques, and focused intentions. The practices of qigong can be classified as martial, medical, or spiritual, but all styles have three things in common: They all involve posture (whether moving or stationary), breathing techniques, and mental focus.

There are a wide variety of qigong practices that can be gentle, as with tai chi, or it can be extremely vigorous with styles, such as kung fu. A unique feature of qigong is the ability to train the mind to direct the body's energy to any part of the body. The practice can relax the mind, muscles, tendons, joints, and inner organs, helping to improve circulation, relieve stress and pain, and restore health.

You can learn qigong at your own pace by taking classes at Learn Qigong Online.* Also check out the Qi Gong Meditation Relaxation* app that includes articles, audios, and videos.

Ballet

Ballet did not begin as an exercise program. It is a form of artistic expression that has its beginnings in the courts of Europe for opera and stage performances. As it has evolved over the years, ballet has become more strenuous and physically demanding, requiring intense focus, discipline, and stamina.

More adults (men and women) are taking recreational ballet classes as a way of keeping fit, flexible, and emotionally engaged. The various components of a typical ballet class, from barre exercises to center work, where you practice dynamic movement combinations, cultivate sustained attention and concentration, as you learn to control the body precisely.

It also requires situational awareness of where the other dancers are and memorization of movement sequences. Even if you are taking a group ballet class, you will find ballet to be an individual, self-focused activity that is a perfect self-care exercise for introverts who want a combination of strength training, coordination, focus, and cardio activity.

In fact, there are many amazing benefits to taking regular ballet classes.

Ballet sculpts and tones your body. The movements taught in ballet class are designed to create long and lean muscles without building up a lot of bulk.

Ballet promotes great posture. To perform the various positions, turns, and combinations in ballet class, your body must be placed in correct posture and alignment. As a result of this specific and repetitive training, you will continue to carry "ballet posture" outside of class.

Ballet promotes strength and flexibility. Ballet requires stretching and extending limbs and muscles and holding these positions using the strength of core muscle groups. Stretching and strength exercises at the ballet barre are an important part of every ballet class. Over time, you will see tremendous improvement in strength and flexibility.

Ballet promotes stamina. Although ballet looks elegant and easy, it requires a great deal of strength and stamina. Repetitive movements, jumps, and dance combinations provide aerobic exercise that gets the heart pumping.

Ballet stimulates mental focus and discipline. To achieve correct positions and proper alignment, you must maintain a high level of concentration and body awareness. Also, the instructor gives a series of movement combinations (in French) that must be quickly memorized and repeated in the classroom. Ballet requires both mental and physical stamina.

Ballet encourages artistic expression. It is an art form, after all, and introverts particularly appreciate the aesthetics of ballet. The technical aspects of ballet require discipline of the body and mind, but the artistic element of dance requires opening your heart and soul. Ballet is a way of expressing and communicating feelings, ideas, and events. A ballet dancer enjoys moving to beautiful and inspiring music and expressing the emotions that the music draws forth.

If you are interested in taking online ballet classes, check out Ballet for Adult Beginners.*

There are many more fitness programs suitable for introverts who prefer solitary exercise or small group classes. When I don't feel like going to my gym, I love to work out at home on my **rebounder, a mini-trampoline** that has a variety of health benefits in addition to a great workout. You can read more about rebounding in an article,* "Rebounding: The Small Trampoline Exercise That's Addictively Fun," on my blog.

You might also consider **ChiRunning**, created by running coach and author Danny Dreyer, and based on movement and mindfulness principles of tai chi. His book, *ChiRunning: A Revolutionary Approach to Effortless, Injury-Free Running*, shows you a new way to run by engaging your core, finding alignment, becoming more relaxed, and blending running with powerful mind-body principles.

Swimming, cycling, spin classes (with your own bike), rowing, walking, and weight training are also good options for you. The important factor is that you find something that suits your personality type and doesn't overwhelm you, while still giving you the workout you need. Override your tendency to sit still and remain in your head all day by finding a fitness routine that suits your introverted nature.

Chapter 3
Create a Well-Care Plan

"Never go to a doctor whose office plants have died."

—Erma Bombeck

I hate going to the doctor, even for routine appointments. It makes me anxious and sets my mind on high alert, wondering whether or not he or she will find "something" that I don't want to deal with. I also dislike calling to make the appointments and dealing with the often brusque and detached office staff.

But the worst part is sitting in the physician's waiting room with the triggering antiseptic smells, elevator music, and other patients nervously waiting to be shuffled back for their own dose of discomfort.

In the past, my dislike of the whole medical thing was strong enough that I would delay appointments far too long, even though I suffered from the guilt and anxiety that procrastination triggers. Eventually, this anxiety would override my resistance, and I would finally set the appointment—but only after tormenting myself for weeks.

I'm sure my introverted nature is the cause of much of my white-coat anxiety, and, as a result, I've had to figure out a way to work around my internal resistance, so I don't jeopardize my health. I know how important it is to have preventative checkups and routine medical exams and procedures. The alternative is burying my head in the sand and hoping that nothing goes wrong—not a smart approach for my long-term health.

Going to the doctor is a special kind of hell for most introverts. In addition to the waiting room misery, you have to endure more foot tapping in a cold exam room, wearing little more than a paper napkin. This is followed by invasive and undignified poking and prodding, all while you attempt to carry on small talk with the doctor or technician.

If you are actually ill and feeling poorly, or you have worrisome symptoms you're having checked out, the entire process is just plain torturous. I don't know about you, but I can't wait to get dressed and make a beeline for the door, leaving all my questions unasked and unanswered.

Doctor's visits are rushed affairs anyway, as most physicians are in a hurry to move on to the next patient. You have to be assertive and even a bit pushy to keep your doc in the room long enough to get all the information and feedback you need. For introverts who are already writhing in discomfort, speaking up assertively as the white coattails are fluttering out the door is no easy task.

With so much going against introverts when it comes to visiting the doctor (or dentist), it's no wonder that we receive substandard healthcare in comparison to extroverts. Knowing this, you must create a self-care plan when it comes to your doctor visits and preventative procedures.

Here are some strategies to make the process more manageable and less daunting.

Appointment Scheduling

- If you have anxiety about doctor's visits or necessary procedures, don't string out your angst like I've done by procrastinating on setting the appointments. Sit and make a list of all of the necessary checkups and procedures you need for the year and determine when you can set the appointments based on your insurance plan.

- Once you have your list, try to schedule all your appointments in one sitting. Take time to put all your doctor (and pharmacy) information on your contact list, including names, email addresses, phone numbers, and any other pertinent information.

- While you're at it, make a list of all your medications and how often you take them, and make a note of any allergies. Put this on your phone so you always have it handy.

- If any of your doctors have online portals, schedule your appointments online to avoid making phone calls. If not, make the calls right away so you don't experience the anxiety of procrastination and avoidance.

- Try to book your appointments for early morning time slots when your doctor hasn't gotten behind schedule. This will minimize your wait time and give you a few more minutes with your doctor before he or she gets slammed with other patients.

- Also avoid appointments on Mondays and Fridays, if possible, as they tend to be the busiest days.

- Definitely avoid booking appointment times that will throw you into rush hour traffic once you leave. After this stressful event, you want to get home as soon as possible to decompress.

- Put all the appointments on your calendar or phone app and set up reminders for a day or two before the appointment so you can mentally prepare.

- If you're going to the doctor because you are ill or have a worrisome symptom, ask your spouse or a friend to make the appointment for you, so you don't have to expend more energy on the phone while dealing with pain or discomfort.

Sitting in the Waiting Room

Nothing is more unnerving than sitting in the waiting room before a doctor's appointment, especially if the room is full of other patients. I tend to arrive at appointments way too early because I think I might be seen early, but this rarely happens.

The better strategy is to arrive just a few minutes before your appointment time, so you don't have to wait as long. Sit in your car until the last minute if necessary.

- While you are in the waiting room, put on headphones and listen to soothing music or an anxiety-reducing podcast.

- Bring an engaging book with you to distract you if you prefer reading.

- Sit away from other people, and even close your eyes so you aren't disrupted by everything around you.

- Practice some slow, meditative breathing if you are feeling anxious, or visualize your time with the doctor going smoothly and calmly.

Asking Questions

- Before you leave the house for your appointment, write down any symptoms, concerns, or questions you want to discuss with your doctor, being as specific as possible.

- Take the list in the exam or procedure room with you, and give it to your doctor as soon as he or she walks in.

- Say something like, "Before you leave the room, these are the concerns and questions I'd like to discuss today." Then you don't have to initiate the conversation as your doctor is trying to wind things up.

- You might think of other questions during the exam, so use the time when your doc reads your list as a trigger to present any additional questions.

- There might be questions you remember after you leave the office, so ask the doctor or a nurse the best way to get questions answered once you are back home.

- You might also consider asking your spouse, partner, or a friend to go to the appointment with you to manage the question-asking part of the appointment and to take notes for you. This is especially useful if your visit relates to a concerning health issue that requires a future procedure, medications, or surgery.

As an introvert, you might feel that your medical needs aren't valid or that you need to pretend or hide how you're feeling. But it's imperative that you avoid this tendency when it comes to your physical, mental, and emotional health. You must speak up if something isn't clear, or you feel your concerns aren't being addressed properly.

If you feel so anxious or uncomfortable in medical settings that you panic and clam up, let your doctor know how you are feeling and that you're having a hard time talking because of anxiety.

Most physicians understand that patients can feel nervous and overwhelmed, and a good healthcare practitioner will slow down and help you feel more comfortable. If not, find another doctor who is more sensitive to your introverted needs.

Chapter 4
Get Plenty of Sleep

"Tired minds don't plan well. Sleep first, plan later."
—Walter Reisch

I frequently have trouble falling asleep quickly, even when I'm exhausted. My body and mind are screaming for some shut-eye, but I can flip around in bed for an hour or more waiting for slumber to descend. Once asleep, I can have vivid and sometimes disturbing dreams that I recall clearly the next day. My mind uses dreams to sort out any worries or challenges I'm dealing with in my waking hours.

I never associated these sleep-related behaviors with my introverted nature until I began research for this book. But I have learned that introversion and sleep are not always a match made in heaven.

Researchers working on behalf of Best Mattress Brand bed company conducted a study* on sleep and personality type. The researchers asked 1,000 people to complete the Myers-Briggs Type Indicator (MBTI) personality test. Then the participants were asked to share information about their sleeping patterns, levels of alertness, and dreams.

The results suggest extroverts are 17.7 percent more satisfied with their levels of energy during waking hours than introverts, and extroverts are also 6.5 percent more satisfied with their ability to sleep through the night than the introverted participants. In comparison, introverts are 14.8 percent less satisfied with the amount they feel alert during waking hours than extroverts.

Because introverts struggle to have a restful night's sleep, they might find it harder to keep their eyes open during the day. According to the study, introverts are 7.7 percent more likely than extroverts to fall asleep during the day when trying to stay awake.

These experiences might be related to the types of dreams that we have. According to the data in the study, "Introverts were more likely to dream of being unable to influence the world around them and dreamed more often of punching without effect. Extroverts, however, dreamed of more active pursuits, such as traveling."

Disturbing dreams, like being lost in the wilderness or being chased but unable to scream, do affect the quality of your sleep and your energy levels throughout the day, according to another study about nightmares.*

Our dreams tend to incorporate aspects of our waking lives in both literal and abstract ways, and they reflect the stress and anxiety we experience during our waking hours. Introverts who are so often in their heads processing information are more prone to sorting out negative events during sleep.

Even though it might not be as restorative and easy for introverts, sleep is a welcome and necessary retreat from the outer world. Because sleep is a specified and acceptable time for shutting down, it is a guilt-free pleasure that requires no engagement or pressure—other than trying to get enough of it.

Knowing how important sleep is to your health and well-being, while recognizing that introverts have less restorative sleep, you need to practice intentional self-care when it comes to your shut-eye.

Here are some strategies you can use to improve your sleep and your energy levels during the day.

1) **Make sleep a priority in your life.** Schedule it as though it's as important as catching an airplane flight or attending a meeting with your supervisor. Ongoing poor sleep affects everything else in your life and can send you spiraling into depression and anxiety.

2) **Go to bed early enough.** If you have to awaken early in the morning, go to bed at a time that allows for a full seven to nine hours of sleep (depending on what makes you feel most rested). Try to stay on a consistent sleep schedule, even on weekends.

3) **Avoid electronics in bed.** Shut down your digital devices before you get into bed. Not only can the news and social media disrupt your ability to fall asleep, but the light from devices is "short-wavelength enriched," meaning it has a higher concentration of blue light than natural light. Blue light affects levels of the sleep-inducing hormone melatonin more than any other wavelength.

4) **Develop a pre-sleep ritual.** Do something relaxing each night before sleep to give your body and brain a signal that it's time to wind down. This might include reading, listening to soft music, or taking a warm bath (which causes your body temperature to drop afterward and makes you sleep).

5) **Take magnesium before bed.** Some studies are showing that taking a magnesium supplement can improve the quality of your sleep. Magnesium plays a role in supporting deep, restorative sleep by maintaining healthy levels of gamma-aminobutyric acid (GABA), a neurotransmitter that promotes sleep. The general dosage is 100–350 mg daily but consult your doctor before taking any supplements.

6) **Make your bedroom conducive to sleep.** That means making it cool (between 60 and 67 degrees Fahrenheit for optimal sleep), dark (use blackout curtains if necessary), and quiet. You might consider putting on a "white noise" app or getting a sound machine.

7) **Avoid caffeine, alcohol, and nicotine before bed.** Try to give a buffer of four to six hours so these substances don't interfere with your sleep.

8) **Don't exercise close to bedtime.** Give yourself at least four hours between the time you exercise and the time you want to go to sleep. But don't use this as an excuse not to exercise.

9) **Don't take long naps during the day.** A short catnap of no more than twenty-five minutes is fine, but more than that will make it hard to fall asleep at bedtime.

10) **Practice meditation.** Meditation will help you manage your racing thoughts and tendency for ruminating, which can disrupt your sleep. It will also reduce stress and anxiety that you might carry to bed with you. If you have trouble falling asleep, try a guided sleep meditation app like Calm* or Headspace.* You'll learn more about meditation in Section 2.

Chapter 5
Pay Attention to Your Body

"Take care of your body. It's the only place you have to live."

—Jim Rohn

As an introvert, you pay a lot of attention to your mind because it's so active, but you might neglect to give the same attention to your body. Beyond getting proper exercise and regular medical attention, you need to listen and respond to what your body is telling you on a daily basis.

Being mindful of your body allows you to be proactive in other forms of physical self-care that facilitate more energy, healing, and balance in your life in general. You already know how profoundly your mind affects your health. Stress, depression, and anxiety can cause a variety of physical symptoms and ailments, some of which can be quite serious and debilitating.

Your body is constantly sending you messages about your well-being, if you pay attention. Something as simple as yawning might not just be a reaction to being tired. It is often a signal that you are dehydrated or even hungry. Heartburn, indigestion, irritable bowel, and headaches could be telling you that you're stressed and dealing with chronic worry.

Are your muscles and joints sore because of your latest workout, or are you sitting too much, carrying extra tension, or dealing with

SELF-CARE FOR INTROVERTS

unresolved emotional issues? Even something like the common cold can be a sign that your immune system is weakened by running on all cylinders.

Often our first response to physical symptoms or messages from our bodies is to mask them. When we're so mentally engaged in reading, writing, working on a project, or contemplating the meaning of life, it's easier to take a pain pill or an antacid medication to calm our physical symptoms. Sometimes this does the trick and relieves the discomfort for good.

But other times medication is just a temporary Band-Aid masking the mental or emotional root cause of your physical reactions. The mind-body connection has been studied for decades, and research* continues to reinforce how profoundly your internal world can express itself through physical symptoms.

Of course, your symptoms might be warning signs of an illness, disease, vitamin deficiency, dehydration, or some other underlying condition. This is another important reason to pay attention to your body and not just hope symptoms will go away.

For introverts, especially those who have health anxiety, focusing on your symptoms might be deeply disconcerting and scary. With your active brain, you might have the tendency to catastrophize and assume the worst-case scenario about every discomfort.

Whether your symptoms are benign or relate to some actual physical problem, it's far better for your *mental health* to find out sooner rather than later. Yes, this means going to the dreaded doctor, but if something is wrong, it needs to be treated. If the symptom is benign or related to your emotional state, you can calm your worst fears and deal with the underlying cause.

If you are tuned into your body every day, you will notice subtle changes and minor discomforts before they become bigger problems or more debilitating afflictions. You can be proactive in tending to both the physical and emotional needs that your body is signaling.

Let's go over some ways you can provide self-care by tuning in to your body.

Perform a Mindful Body Scan

In the morning, before you've eaten anything or started moving around, close your eyes and mentally scan your entire body. Begin at your toes, slowly moving up to all of your limbs, your torso, your neck, back, and head. Be sure to notice your muscles, joints, and organs. Pay attention to any areas of discomfort, pain, tension, or malaise.

As you encounter an area of discomfort, breath into it, and ask yourself what is going on to cause this sensation. Sit quietly for a moment and see what comes up for you. You might not get an answer immediately, but you have planted the seed of attention and awareness, which can do its work in your subconscious mind, revealing an answer at a later time.

In future body scans, return to those areas of discomfort that seem unexplainable or have no discernible cause. Notice whether the feeling has changed—gotten better, gotten worse, or disappeared. Some of these pains are just physical blips that don't require special action or attention.

However, during your scan, you might get an inkling about the cause of your discomfort, and if so, mentally explore this further.

If stress or sadness seems to be the culprit, ask yourself why you are feeling this way and what you need to do to relieve or treat these emotions.

Once you identify that something in your internal world is causing symptoms, you might feel relieved or even emotional about your discovery. Allow whatever feelings come up to flow through you without getting too attached to them.

Your attention to your body might reveal some practical actions you need to take. If you have a headache, you might discern you need to drink more water. If your neck is cramping, your pillow might be too thick. Taking time for this body scan helps you make the slight tweaks to your daily decisions that can make you feel more energetic and comfortable.

You might consider adding an evening body scan to your daily routine to see how your symptoms have changed or whether stress from your day has contributed to new physical discomforts. At least you will become intimately familiar with your body and how it functions and responds. You will learn to fine-tune your self-care to enhance your physical well-being.

Get Regular Guilt-Free Massages

Introverts are more sensitive to light, noise, and especially people. You become easily overstimulated, even being around your own family and children for too long. Your family often needs more of you than you can easily tolerate, making you feel claustrophobic from the demands on your psyche.

Of course, this makes you feel guilty and stressed because you think you *should* be more available, attentive, and enthusiastic with those you care about. You feel derelict hiding out in your room with the door closed while your family searches the house for you.

Do they view you as selfish or unloving because of your need for alone time to recharge? This fear can keep you from setting the boundaries that your personality type so desperately needs.

That's why getting massages is so valuable for introverts. You get to leave the house, get away from others, and retreat to a sanctuary where the psychological volume is turned down.

You also get a physical treatment that relieves the stress and emotional overwhelm you often feel as a result of your introverted nature. If you are a highly sensitive introvert (something we'll discuss more in Section 2), you might find massage an almost spiritual experience because of your extra sensitivity to physical touch.

There are many other benefits to getting regular massages that will help you justify this level of self-care to yourself and your family. Many research studies* confirm that massage helps reduce chronic pain, decreases depression and anxiety, promotes relaxation, and reduces symptoms associated with fibromyalgia. Massage also calms the nervous system and improves blood and lymphatic circulation.

As beneficial as massage is, you still might find yourself avoiding it. Because of the self-imposed guilt trips we introverts tend to take, you might feel it's too indulgent to get massages, concerned that others will view you as extra needy or high maintenance.

Introverts have a particularly difficult time justifying self-care and might hold the false belief that receiving a massage is too luxurious and the "wrong" way to spend time and money. But as deep thinkers, introverts also recognize on some level that this mindset isn't productive, and that self-care is especially important for introverts.

Introverts also shy away from getting massages for the same reason they avoid going to the doctor. You don't want someone up in your space while you're in a state of partial undress. And you especially don't want to be trapped in a small, dark room with someone who is chattering away while you're trying to escape and sink into the pleasure of peaceful alone time.

But you can control the massage environment more than you might think. The important goal is to find a massage therapist you trust, who knows you're an introvert and that you need a "no chit-chat" policy during your sessions.

From my personal experience, most therapists will get the message if they start talking and receive a monosyllabic response in return. But you can be proactive at the beginning of a massage by saying, "Please ask me any questions before we get started, because I prefer a quiet massage experience."

Start by asking your friends for recommendations or look online, on a site like Angie's List, for reviews of spas and massage therapists near you. Then interview several therapists to learn about their massage style, level of pressure, the physical space of the massage room, and the kind of music they play. A good massage therapist will ask you about your preferences and what your goals are with massage.

Making massage a regular part of your schedule is important if it is going to be included in your self-care plan. A yearly massage is relaxing and a nice treat, but it can't undo years of muscle tension or help you manage stress. Depending on the amount you exercise and your stress levels, consider beginning with once a week or twice a month. Then cut back to monthly sessions to maintain the health of your muscle tissue.

Of course, your budget might determine how often you can get a massage. A massage at a spa can range from $70 to over $100 for an hour, plus you will need to add a 15–20 percent tip. A private practitioner generally charges less, somewhere between $60 and $90 an hour.

A more affordable option is Massage Envy, a franchise with 1,200 locations in 49 states, which offers more no-frills, monthly massage. You can try it out for an introductory price ($55–$75), and then sign up for a monthly massage ranging from $65 to $85 a month, depending on the market.

If you can't afford to get a massage, give yourself one. First, warm your body in a hot bath or apply a heating pad to the areas of the body you're massaging. Rub your skin with massage oil or a natural oil, like coconut, grapeseed, or raw sesame oil. Use a fascia massager (a massage stick roller) to break up tight fascia tissue around your muscles.

If you are especially tight throughout the week, you can do this for your shoulders, neck, and jaw a few times a week. Then make Saturdays or Sundays your day for whole body massage using the fascia tool.

Stand and Move Frequently

Do a quick online search of "best careers for introverts," and you'll see that more than half the jobs listed are some form of desk job—accounting, software developer, writer, court reporter, social media manager, etc.

There are certainly plenty of suitable jobs for introverts that keep you more on your feet, but many of you reading this book can relate to the fact that we spend a lot of time sitting, whether at work or in our personal lives. We're the people who want to come home after work and curl up with a good book or watch a movie. You won't often find us at the local bar with coworkers or going out dancing to blow off steam.

The average office worker sits for about ten hours a day, including time at work and at home. In fact, the World Health Organization estimates that 95 percent of the adult population in the world is inactive, not meeting the minimum recommendations of thirty minutes of moderate to intense physical activity five times a week.

If you recognize yourself as more of a "sitter" than someone who likes to be up moving around most of the day, then you need to pay particular attention to this self-care strategy.

Research links sitting for long periods (whether at work, in front of the TV, or in your car) with obesity, cardiovascular disease, and cancer. The research reveals that men who sit six hours or more a day have a death rate 20 percent higher than men who sit for three hours or less. And alarmingly, for women, it's 40 percent higher.

Even if you spend some time every week at the gym or exercising, it doesn't offset the negative impact of extended sitting. The only solution is to get off your butt to move around more in general.

Before you worry that you need to get a new job that keeps you on your feet, you should know that working all day standing up isn't the solution either. Prolonged standing also has health risks, like carotid atherosclerosis (a disease of the arteries), which increase ninefold due to the extra weight on your circulatory system.

You're also more likely to get varicose veins, which aren't attractive and cause all sorts of complications. Plus, if you stand for long periods, your knees start to ache, your feet start to feel numb, and it can just get uncomfortable.

A 2015 article* in *The Washington Post* clarifies exactly how much sitting and standing we should be doing for optimal health.

According to the expert statement released in the British Journal of Sports Medicine, Americans should begin to stand, move and take breaks for at least two out of eight hours at work. Then, Americans should gradually work up to spending at least half of your eight-hour work day in what researchers call these "light-intensity activities."

So what's the solution? The answer is creating a personalized plan that includes some sitting, some standing, and lots of moving around. If you work at a desk job, you can consider a plan like this.

- Work for an hour or so standing.
- Walk around or move for fifteen minutes.
- Work for an hour or so sitting.
- Get up and move around again for fifteen minutes.

- Go back to standing.
- Repeat the switch between sitting, standing, and moving all day.
- Find time for thirty to forty-five minutes of daily cardio.

You might need to set a timer on your smartphone or watch to help you remember to stay on track with this plan. But there are other ways you can ensure you're moving around more so that you don't jeopardize your health and shorten your lifespan.

- Rather than texting or emailing someone at work, walk to his or her office to talk instead.
- Take the stairs rather than the elevator.
- Stand and pace whenever you are on the phone.
- Don't eat your lunch at your desk—walk to a restaurant or a park.
- Pace when you are brainstorming, which can actually stimulate your creativity.
- When you hit that 3:00 p.m. slump at work, go outside and take a walk to re-energize, rather than grabbing a cup of coffee.
- At home when watching television, get up during commercials and march in place or do jumping jacks.
- If you work from home, consider getting a standing desk or a treadmill desk. If you can't afford a treadmill desk, you can hack your own* by stacking a small table on your desk and purchasing an inexpensive treadmill from Amazon.
- If you have been sitting for a long time, be sure to include stretching as part of your movement plan. Tight hips and

inactive glutes can hinder your physical performance in a variety of activities.

What's critical here is that you do *something* to keep yourself moving throughout the day, even at home when you just want to crash on the couch for the evening. Find ways to "gamify" your movement and challenge yourself to slowly increase your moving time and decrease your sitting time throughout the day. Take care of your health by adding this change to your self-care routine.

Hydrate Consistently

Drinking more water should be a goal for everyone, not just introverts. But it is an especially valuable self-care tool for introverts who often don't pay enough attention to their body's need for hydration.

An average guideline is to drink six to eight, 8-ounce glasses of water a day or about 2 liters. If you are exercising, breastfeeding, or ill with the flu or a urinary tract infection, you'll need to drink more.

Water is the best way to hydrate, but if you can't stomach the idea of downing eight glasses a day, you can reach this goal by drinking juices and eating water-rich foods such as salads, fruit, and applesauce. Just remember, juices often have a high sugar and calorie content.

If you're not drinking the recommended daily amount of water, there are several good reasons that you, as an introvert, should change your ways.

1) You're already susceptible to not getting enough sleep and feeling tired and distracted during the day. Staying hydrated maintains your energy levels because it keeps your muscles energized. Fatigue or low energy is often caused by dehydration, so staying hydrated will help you feel more energized.

2) You'll also be more productive and clear-headed when you drink enough water, as even mild dehydration can cause disorientation, dizziness, and fuzzy thinking. Dehydration is also known to cause headaches and difficulty concentrating, which further hampers your productivity.

3) You're also more susceptible to stress than your extroverted friends, and there's a surprising correlation between staying hydrated and your mood. A study published in the British Journal of Nutrition* found that male participants experienced fatigue, tension, and anxiety when dehydrated. Even being mildly dehydrated can affect your mood, energy level, and ability to think clearly, according to studies conducted at the University of Connecticut's Human Performance Laboratory.*

4) One of the symptoms of chronic dehydration can be depression (something introverts are susceptible to), and there are several ways dehydration and depression are linked. Depression is connected to insufficient levels of serotonin, the neurotransmitter that largely determines mood. Dehydration reduces these serotonin levels.

An amino acid called tryptophan is converted to serotonin in your brain, and an adequate amount of water is necessary for tryptophan to be carried across the blood-brain barrier.

Dehydration limits the amount of tryptophan available to the brain, thus reducing serotonin levels.

Stress is a significant factor leading to depression. When you feel stressed, your adrenal glands produce more of the stress hormone cortisol. With chronic stress, these glands can become exhausted.

Not only can dehydration cause stress and depression, but stress can also cause dehydration. Your adrenal glands make aldosterone, a hormone that helps to regulate your body's fluid and electrolyte levels. As adrenal fatigue gets worse, the production of aldosterone drops, triggering dehydration and low electrolytes.

In addition to affecting your energy levels, ability to concentrate, and your mood, all significant factors for introverts, hydrating your body has many other valuable benefits, including the following.

- Making your skin suppler and more elastic. (Most internal water is lost through the skin.)
- Maintaining body-fluid balance, which is important for saliva production and maintaining body temperature.
- Keeping your kidneys functioning properly.
- Maintaining normal bowel movements.
- Promoting cardiovascular health by maintaining your blood volume.
- Helping your muscles and joints work better.

If you don't know whether or not you are dehydrated, your body gives you some fairly strong indicators that you need to pay attention to.

Increased thirst and a dry or sticky mouth: If you are thirsty, you're already dehydrated.

Dark urine: If your urine is straw-colored or light yellow, you are hydrated. Dark urine means you need to up your water intake.

Shriveled and dry skin: If you are dehydrated your skin will appear dry and will lack elasticity and won't bounce back if you pinch it.

Signs of fatigue, confusion, or anger: Feeling tired or out of sorts? You could be running on empty when it comes to your water tank.

Dry eyes or blurred vision: This is another sign that your body is craving water.

Headaches or disorientation: Dehydration can cause headaches and even migraines and can make you feel lightheaded or delirious.

Muscle cramping: This is because of the loss of water and salt in the body, especially after exercising.

Lack of sweat: This is a serious sign of dehydration and could mean your body is in serious need of water. (This can also be a sign of overheating or heat stroke.)

You want to be proactive about staying hydrated, so you don't experience these symptoms or the mental and emotional issues that dehydration can cause. You might not naturally think about hydrating all day, but there are several simple ways you can make this a daily self-care habit.

1) **Change your mindset.** If you have a prized garden or a favorite houseplant, you stay on top of watering it. You wouldn't forget to fill your beloved pet's water bowl. Your body needs water just like every other living thing, and

you need to treat your body with loving care. Make getting enough water a priority.

2) **Keep a water bottle nearby.** Find a sturdy, glass, stainless steel, or BPA-free 2-liter water bottle and keep it with you next to your desk and in your car. Drink from it all day— you'll know you've gotten your daily dose of water when the bottle is empty.

3) **Jazz up your water.** If you hate the taste of plain water, add a slice of lemon or lime to give it more flavor. Or try a flavored carbonated water (without added sugar or sugar substitutes), which hydrates you just as well as plain water.

4) **Drink water after a trigger.** I make a habit of drinking a glass of water after I use the restroom throughout the day. You can use other triggers to remind you to drink, like every time you go to the sink or stand up.

5) **Substitute water for caffeinated drinks.** If you drink a lot of caffeinated drinks throughout the day, you'll need even more water. Consider substituting a glass of water for one or two of those drinks.

6) **Drink water when you're hungry.** Often, we think we're hungry when we are really thirsty. Real hunger won't be satisfied by drinking water. Drinking a glass of water before you eat can make you feel fuller, which can contribute to healthy weight loss.

7) **Drink water before, during, and after exercise.** You need extra water when you work out (about every ten to twenty minutes) to stay hydrated.

8) **Don't go crazy.** Don't start downing water without paying attention to how much you're consuming. Too much water

can lead to hyponatremia, when excess water in our bodies dilutes the sodium content of our blood.

Drinking enough water during the day might feel like more of a chore rather than a self-care technique. But self-care isn't just giving yourself a little TLC—it's also preventative care. Introverts must be especially mindful of the behaviors and choices that will help them feel their best and thrive, both at work and in their personal lives. So go fill your glass and drink up!

Chapter 6
The Introvert Diet

"Food is not just eating energy. It's an experience."

—Guy Fieri

Have you noticed that you have special dietary needs—foods that help you feel more healthy, energetic, and emotionally balanced? Maybe you experience uncomfortable symptoms, such as irritable bowel, headaches, anxiety, skin disorders, and low energy, that seem to be associated with certain foods and beverages.

Does the trait of introversion have something to do with these diet sensitivities? The research on the connection is thin, but anecdotal evidence suggests that there's a connection between your introverted personality traits and the way you respond to the foods you eat and the beverages you consume.

There is certainly evidence to show that specific foods, beverages, and chemicals can trigger symptoms of anxiety and depression, mood disorders that are common with introverts. Your introversion might not make you sensitive to certain foods, but introversion makes you more susceptible to mood reactions that foods can also trigger.

Many introverts identify as "highly sensitive people," and there is a science-backed connection between sensitive people and food tolerance. Highly sensitive people (HSPs) can be triggered by certain chemicals and foods, such as caffeine, refined sugar, processed foods, additives, and dairy. HSPs are also known to have sophisticated, subtle pallets and even a strong distaste for certain foods that other nonsensitives can tolerate.

Although not all introverts are highly sensitive people, the majority of HSPs (about 70 percent) are introverts, according to research by Dr. Elaine Aron, a pioneer in researching highly sensitive people. We'll discuss HSPs in more detail in Section 2, but for now it's important to be aware of the relationship between introversion and HSPs, and how it can affect your tolerance for certain foods.

If you're a highly sensitive introvert like me, you are keenly aware of being hypersensitive to certain foods, although you might not have associated your reactions to your personality traits.

Like many HSPs, I have a low tolerance for caffeine. One cup of coffee makes me want to jump out of my skin and leaves me anxious and agitated for hours. You might have this same reaction to caffeine or to other foods and chemicals because of your more sensitive nature.

The Introvert's Value-Driven Diet

Some introverts follow a strict diet based on their personal values without as much regard to how the foods make them feel. As deep thinkers who are guided by internal experiences, many introverts carefully (even obsessively) deliberate over the foods they choose to eat, making sure to consider how their food choices align with their values.

They create a conscious diet that can include a variety of factors, such as cruelty to animals, impact on the environment, longevity, and disease prevention. In fact, sensitive, empathic introverts can feel deep discomfort and aversion to eating meat or animal products because of their intense compassion for animals.

Introverts also tend to think more about the consequences of what they are putting in their mouths, more so than the average person. Because you are more likely to delve deep into topics that interest you, diet and nutrition might be high on the list, given your propensity for making well-considered decisions.

You are less impulsive about eating whatever you crave, and more likely to pause and consider future weight gain or heart disease before ordering that burger and fries.

Having a values-driven diet can give you a deep sense of satisfaction and confidence, knowing that you've applied research, contemplation, and commitment to something that you believe is important. Being disciplined with that commitment only adds to your positive feelings about yourself and your choices.

But does a values-driven diet work for every introvert? Not necessarily.

How to Determine Your Ideal Diet

There is no one perfect diet that works for all introverts, even highly sensitive introverts. The best diet for you is the one that makes you feel the best physically, mentally, and emotionally.

And even though your value system might prevent you from eating certain foods and choosing others, if these choices make you feel sluggish, tired, anxious, uncomfortable, or ill, then you might want to reexamine your choices. You might have to decide between a body-driven diet and a values-driven diet related to certain foods.

I tried eating a vegetarian diet for several months for ethical and health reasons, only to feel irritable, constantly hungry, and tired. Once I added fish and chicken back into my diet, I felt much better and had more energy. My quality of life, which is an important value for me, trumped my desire to be a vegetarian.

These decisions are personal and often emotionally charged, and it might require some soul-searching and trial and error to determine your own ideal diet. It's important to listen to the wisdom of your body, even if it's sometimes in conflict with the wisdom of your mind.

Your reactions and sensitives to certain foods could well have nothing to do with your personality and be related to allergies or other intolerances that affect introverts and extroverts alike. But as an introvert who is already prone to depression and anxiety and often avoids going to the doctor, you need to pay careful attention to your diet and how your body responds to foods.

Food allergies and intolerances can lead to a host of physical problems (everything from headaches, skin disorders, and gut problems to more serious reactions like immune system problems) that will also affect your mental health. With all these considerations, how can you choose the best diet for your body?

You might begin by asking yourself these questions.

- What uncomfortable physical symptoms do I notice regularly? (These might include stomach and intestinal problems, bloating, skin irritations and rashes, headaches, yeast infections, anxiety, depression, fatigue, irritability, congestion, cravings, inability to concentrate, and sleep problems.)

- Do these symptoms occur most often after eating (or drinking) or within a few hours of eating?

- If I'm not sure about a food connection, do I have an inkling or sense that maybe a food or beverage is causing my symptoms?

- When I avoid certain foods or beverages, do I notice any symptoms dissipating or going away entirely?

- If there a food group I've given up, could the absence of that food contribute to my physical or emotional symptoms?

- What have I recently eaten when I'm feeling really good and energetic?

If you have an inkling about a food or drink that might be causing your symptoms, consider eliminating it for a while to see if the symptoms go away. Keep a journal and write down what you are eating, what you are eliminating, and how you feel every day. Eliminate just one food at a time so you'll know exactly what is or isn't causing your symptoms. Reintroduce these foods slowly.

Likely Food Culprits

Trigger foods: Foods that can trigger a sensitive system include wheat, dairy, beans and legumes, and complex grains. Other foods can cause inflammation and can be difficult to digest, including cruciferous vegetables (like broccoli, cauliflower, celery, and asparagus) and aromatics (like garlic and onions). Some people also have trouble with nightshades, like eggplant and tomatoes. Other common food sensitivities include peanuts, soy, seafood, and tree nuts.

Caffeine: Caffeine is a stimulant and can make you anxious and jittery, especially if you're highly sensitive. If you are already stressed and anxious, you should definitely cut back on caffeinated beverages.

Alcohol: Alcohol is a depressant and is known to disrupt sleep, so if you are prone to depression or having sleep problems, consider cutting back or avoiding alcohol altogether.

Sugar: Sugar (which is in alcohol and in so many foods) also has a connection to depression. A 2015 study* of postmenopausal women demonstrated that an increase in added sugars in their diet was associated with an increased likelihood of depression.

Aspartame: This common ingredient in diet sodas blocks the production of the neurotransmitter serotonin (the calming brain chemical), which can lead to headaches, insomnia, and changes in mood.

Fast Food: I'm sure you know the myriad health reasons to avoid fast food, but you might not know that if eaten regularly, fast foods can make you depressed. According to a 2012 study* in the journal *Public Health Nutrition,* people who eat fast food are 51 percent more likely to develop depression than those who don't.

Foods to Prioritize

There are some diet choices you can make with reasonable confidence, knowing you are treating your body and mind well (unless you have allergies to any of these). Many of these foods can help you manage stress, anxiety, and feelings of depression. Here are a few you might want to consider.

Add probiotic foods to your diet. A study* published in August 2015 in the journal *Psychiatry Research* found a link between consuming probiotic foods (like pickles, sauerkraut, and kefir) and a lowering of social anxiety. A new study* published in 2017 in the *Annals of General Psychiatry* linked probiotics with improving symptoms of major depressive disorder, by either decreasing inflammation in the body or by increasing the availability of serotonin.

Choose foods with omega-3 fatty acids. An Ohio State University College of Medicine study* showed that omega-3 fatty acids are especially good for reducing anxiety symptoms. This nutrient is found in fatty fish, like wild salmon, flaxseed, walnuts, and chia seeds. Other studies* have found that people who consume omega-3s regularly are less likely to be depressed. In addition to these mental health benefits, omega-3s have a variety of other benefits from fighting inflammation to reducing risk factors for heart disease.

Eat more high antioxidant foods. Antioxidants protect the brain against free radicals that lead to inflammation, which can impair neurotransmitter production. Anxiety symptoms are linked with a lower antioxidant state.

The ten foods with the highest amount of antioxidants include the following.

- Goji berries
- Wild blueberries
- Dark chocolate
- Pecans
- Artichoke (boiled)
- Elderberries
- Kidney beans
- Cranberries
- Blackberries
- Cilantro

Other high antioxidant foods include tomatoes, carrots, pumpkin seeds, sweet potatoes, pomegranates, strawberries, kale, broccoli, grapes or red wine, squash, and wild-caught salmon.

Add More Magnesium-Rich Foods to Your Diet

Magnesium is a mineral that is calming and can induce relaxation. Research* underscores that magnesium can help treat mental health problems. According to another study,* inadequate magnesium reduces levels of the mood-determining neurotransmitter serotonin.

Reinforcing this link, researchers found that antidepressants tend to increase magnesium in the brain. Magnesium can be found in foods such as eggs, greens (spinach and Swiss chard), legumes, nuts, seeds, and avocados.

Eat Foods Rich in Vitamin B

Vitamin B also has a positive effect on the nervous system and has been shown to decrease feelings of anxiety. Deficiencies in vitamin B have been linked to anxiety disorders.

According to Penn State Hershey Medical Center, a study* found that vitamin B6 helps the body make several mood-influencing neurotransmitters, including serotonin. A Miller School of Medicine at the University of Miami study* revealed that adults with depression had fewer depressive and anxious symptoms after two months of taking a vitamin B complex.

Some of the best foods for vitamin B include eggs, brewer's yeast, lentils, split peas, black beans, spinach, mushrooms, salmon, pine nuts, sunflower seeds, collard greens, soybeans, and beef liver.

Here are some other diet self-care ideas to consider.

- If you are a vegetarian and experience fatigue or low energy, consider adding small amounts of fish to your diet or speak with your doctor about a supplement that might help you feel better if you want to remain a vegetarian.

- Try to eat in a calm, stress-free environment, as the stress hormone cortisol can shut down the digestive process. Don't eat while watching the news or an agitating television program. Try not to have heated conversations during your meals. Be more mindful of what you are eating, slowing down enough to savor the flavors and textures of your food.

- Liquid dilutes the digestive juices of your stomach, making your body work harder to digest your food, so drink small amounts with your meals. Then wait at least thirty minutes after a meal to drink more.

- Rather than jumping up as soon as you're done eating, allow some time when you've finished your meal to sit and relax so your body can do the work of digestion.

- Eat at regular times each day to put your digestion on a predictable schedule that allows you a better chance of digesting fully.

Ultimately, the best diet for you is the one that makes you feel the best. If you are highly sensitive, have sleep difficulties, have a tendency toward depression or anxiety, or you just notice that certain foods disagree with you, pay attention and adjust your diet accordingly.

If you don't notice any unpleasant physical or emotional symptoms related to what you consume, but you have strong values about your food choices, honor your values and your commitment to them by being more mindful of what you eat on a daily basis.

Proper self-care with your diet means paying attention, listening to your body, contemplating your priorities, and finding the best balance that works for you.

Chapter 7
Body and Skin Care Rituals

"Invest in your skin. It is going to represent you for a very long time."
—Linden Tyler

When my children were young, there were evenings when I fell asleep with a full face of makeup, too exhausted to clean my face properly before bed. But I hated the feeling of waking up with yesterday's makeup, so I decided to begin my skin care routine earlier in the evening rather than doing another load of laundry or some other chore.

Having that brief time to myself, while my kids were playing or doing homework, gave me the breather I needed to calmly get them to bed and feel better about my own skin and body care hygiene.

Your body and skin care routine shouldn't be a chore but rather a satisfying ritual that you find soothing and therapeutic. The word "ritual" itself suggests something ceremonial, spiritual, and meaningful. If you focus on your actions and the rituals, they aren't just a means to an end, they are deeply valuable on their own. And, of course, as introverts, we are always seeking more meaning and purpose behind our actions.

Taking care of your skin, one of the largest organs of the human body, is purpose enough for ritualizing this part of your self-care.

Your skin works hard to protect your body from harmful elements and taking regular care of your skin can protect you from skin issues in the future. Having a regular skin care routine will also help you look and feel better, boosting your confidence and self-esteem—for men and women.

If you're an introverted man who doesn't regularly practice any kind of skin care routine other than washing your face and shaving, you might want to keep reading. Men have special skin care needs, just like women—especially if they want to avoid signs of aging, acne, dryness, and other skin issues.

Unfortunately, this area of self-care is often neglected. Life is so hectic and demanding that we feel lucky to splash some water on our faces and brush our teeth before falling into bed. This is especially true if you have children who seem to need your undivided attention until the moment your head hits the pillow.

But making the time to take care of your skin (on your face and body) can improve your overall well-being and perhaps fill your tank enough to have more energy and presence of mind to better tend to the needs of your family. Whether you are putting on a facial mask before taking a long and relaxing bath, or you're taking the time to exfoliate before you begin your day, having a peaceful ritual can promote relaxation and reduce stress.

Body and skin care rituals are typically solitary activities that provide the quiet time you crave while keeping you out of your overactive mind. Nighttime rituals also set you up for the restful night's sleep introverts need to recharge themselves.

Rather than zoning out in front of the TV or unwinding with one too many adult beverages, use that time after a long day at work to do something good for your body and mind. Guys, it might feel awkward to slosh around in the tub while wearing a clay mask, but, hey, you're an introvert, so who's going to see you? You can still watch your favorite game or enjoy a drink while hydrating your skin.

Doing anything that boosts your mood and makes you feel peaceful and happy can have a positive impact on your well-being. Says Mason Currey, author of *Daily Rituals: How Artists Work*, "A solid routine fosters a well-worn groove for one's mental energies and helps stave off the tyranny of moods" (page 1).

When you have a daily skin care ritual, you create one chunk of time you can look forward to when you aren't turned inward, but rather you're focused on giving yourself a little TLC.

Here are some body and skin care rituals that are great for introverts.

Take Long, Soothing Baths

Taking a long bath is one of the best ways to relax, and it can also be great for your skin, if you add some nourishing oils. Recent studies* have also shown that taking a hot bath burns as many calories as a thirty-minute walk. That's quite a bonus for introverts who might prefer bathing to walking!

- Before you slip into your liquid, calorie-reduction tub, make sure your bathroom is clean, so you create the proper environment for relaxation. A big factor in stress reduction is getting rid of clutter and being in a clean and peaceful environment.

- If you want to create a spa-like setting, dim the lights, put on some relaxing music (try the Shaman's Dream station on

Pandora), and light scented candles around the tub. Have some clean, fluffy towels nearby and roll a smaller towel to put under your neck.

- Put all your face and body cleansing items and anything else you might want (a book, glass of wine, cup of tea, etc.) on a tray that you can easily reach while bathing.

- When you're running your bath, be sure the water is warm, but not uncomfortably hot. You don't want to dry out or damage your skin by immersing yourself in water that could cook a lobster!

- Make this bathing ritual a mindfulness experience. As you get undressed, listen to the sounds of the water running. Gently enter the tub, submerging yourself in the warm, healing water. Breathe deeply and take in the soothing aromas of the candles and the water.

To help make your bath more relaxing, add some soothing oils or bath salts to the water. Jillee Nystul, blogger and founder of the site "One Good Thing," has a recipe* for an intoxicating eucalyptus mint bath oil.

To make this oil, follow these instructions.

- Mix twenty drops of eucalyptus essential oil with ten drops of peppermint essential oil.

- Add this mixture to 2–3 ounces of a carrier oil (like almond, coconut, or grapeseed oil) in a small bottle or jar.

- Shake the mixture well before each use so separation doesn't occur.

- Add a tablespoon of the mixture to your bath as you're running the water.

Using this bath oil with some Epsom salt will help relax your muscles and soothe your sore body if you have had a long and exhausting day.

Another great option for a calming bath is to create a rose milk bath. Rose oil has natural anti-inflammatory and antibacterial properties. Rose oil is also moisturizing for your skin and can keep it from becoming red or irritated.

To make a rose bath, add the following to your bath.

- Four to six drops of rose essential oil
- 1½ cups of powdered milk
- ½ cup of Epsom salt
- ¼ cup of dried rose petals

Of course, you can purchase a variety of bath oils, bath bombs, and soaks, but part of the enjoyment of this ritual might be creating your own and blending essential oils that you find the most soothing, relaxing, and aromatic. More on essential oils below.

When you get out of the tub, pat yourself dry and apply body oil or lotion from face to toe. Wrap yourself in a comfy robe or pajamas and try to maintain your relaxed state until it's time for bed.

Practice an Evening Skin Care Routine

Because your nights are probably a lot less rushed than your mornings, this is a perfect time to focus some extra attention on your skin. You'll feel better knowing that your skin is going to get the attention it deserves, and the evening is the best time to get rid of environmental pollutants, dirt, and makeup that accumulate on your face all day.

The first thing any man or woman needs to do when considering a skin care ritual is to figure out their skin type. Your skin is either normal, oily, dry, combination, or aging.

- If your skin is normal, it means that your skin rarely gets oily during the day and acne is not a problem for you.
- Oily skin means that you do start to feel greasy during the day and your skin is prone to breakouts.
- Dry or sensitive skin often feels tight and can get irritated.
- Combination skin means that some parts of your face tend to be oily (usually the T-zone) while your cheeks typically remain dry.
- Aging skin has age spots, wrinkles, and looks weathered.

Figure out which skin type best matches yours before choosing products to use during your routine. A good evening skin care routine will involve cleansing, exfoliating, smoothing on a mask, and adding hydration to your skin.

One of the most important things you can do for the health of your skin is using a good cleanser to remove makeup and get all the dirt and oil off your skin.

In fact, each night you sleep with your makeup on, your pores get increasingly clogged, and you set yourself up for skin breakouts and aggravation. It can also damage your skin over time to regularly leave the chemicals in makeup sitting on your face.

Find a good cleanser that is right for your skin type and use it twice a day. One of the most commonly recommended cleansers for all skin types is Cetaphil Gentle Skin Cleanser which you can buy at most drugstores or online.

After cleansing, exfoliation helps shed dead skin cells and generate new ones. If your old skin cells start to build up on your skin's surface, it can leave your skin looking and feeling dull, dry, and rough. Also, the build-up of dead skin cells might lead to excess oil and clogged pores, which can cause blemishes and acne.

Using a face mask can be a valuable part of a skin care ritual, although you might want to use a mask only a few times a week rather than daily. Masks are easy to apply and great at delivering positive results. They can hydrate skin, remove excess oil, help shrink your pores, and help remove impurities.

When your skin is well-hydrated, it is more plump and resilient. It's important to hydrate the skin both from the inside and the outside. You should drink a lot of water throughout the day and apply a high-quality moisturizer at night. This will help prevent wrinkles and keep your skin looking healthy and vibrant.

Men are not excused from taking care of their skin, even though it might seem like a girls-only activity. Guys, use a facial cleanser to wash your face twice a day and exfoliate between one and three times each week before you shave. This helps prevent ingrown hairs and irritation.

Men also need to hydrate their skin, so it doesn't lose its elasticity. Apply a men's moisturizer after washing your face, and don't forget to moisturize your eyes and forehead. This is even important if you tend to have oily skin.

Men also need to use preventative measures to keep their skin healthy and free from sun damage. This means using at least an SPF 15 on all parts of your exposed skin every day.

Try Dry Brushing

Dry brushing is a meditative and relaxing process for introverts that is becoming increasingly popular—even popping up as an offering on spa menus. It has several potential benefits, such as giving you smoother skin, exfoliation, and cleaning out your pores. It also feels really good, even though you'd think rubbing a dry brush over your skin might be a form of self-flagellation.

However, the key is having the right brush. Choose a natural bristle brush with a long handle so you can reach your entire back and brush the bottoms of your feet and the backs of your legs.

Start with a gentle brush to get your skin used to the feeling, and then you can work up to a firmer brush if you wish. You can find dual-head brushes that have harder bristles on one side for exfoliation and softer bristles on the other to increase blood flow and for more sensitive areas.

Take some time each morning to dry brush before you get in the shower. Start by brushing the bottoms of your feet and work your way up your legs. Brush each section of your body about ten times, starting gently and gradually increasing the pressure.

Move on to your arms, beginning with your palms and brushing up your arms toward your heart. When you are brushing your stomach, use a gentler brush and move it in a circular, clockwise motion. Avoid sensitive or damaged skin altogether.

Try this out to see if you enjoy it. Experts have mixed opinions on the effectiveness of dry brushing for some claims (like clearing out toxins and banishing cellulite), but it is a relaxing activity that helps exfoliate and brighten your skin.

Use Aromatherapy with Essential Oils

Do certain smells create a mood and help you feel calm and peaceful? Do you find yourself more sensitive to smells and aware of how they affect your state of mind? If you're a highly sensitive introvert, some smells might trigger a migraine or make you nauseous. But perhaps the aroma of certain essential oils has a more positive effect, helping you feel centered and serene after a highly stimulating day.

Essential oils are known to provide a variety of benefits, both physical and emotional. Research is somewhat limited on the effectiveness of aromatherapy—the therapeutic use of essential oils. However, some studies* have shown that aromatherapy does provide valuable benefits, including relief from anxiety and depression and improved sleep.

You can use essential oils to complement other self-care rituals and activities to create a soothing, relaxing environment enhanced by your favorite aromas. I particularly love the smell of lavender, mainly because it reminds me of being in a spa and signals relaxation.

Aromatherapy works by stimulating the smell receptors in the nose. These receptors send messages through the nervous system to the limbic system, which is the part of the brain that controls emotions. This is good news if you are an introvert who is prone to depression and has sleep problems, as essential oils can be a complementary therapy for people with these health concerns.

Four great essential oils* for introverts include bergamot, lavender, clary sage, and ylang-ylang.

Bergamot essential oil can be used as a massage oil for stress relief and overall relaxation. Studies have shown that bergamot can also reduce blood pressure and heart rate.

Lavender essential oil is often used for treating symptoms of anxiety, depression, restlessness, and disturbed sleep—improving quality and quantity of sleep by promoting relaxation.

Clary sage essential oil is known to help manage symptoms of depression and reduce anxiety. Research shows that clary sage oil is found to be effective in controlling cortisol levels (the stress hormone) in women.

Ylang-ylang has a warm and soothing scent that can be used for reducing stress. The fragrance is intensely intoxicating, sweet, floral, and slightly spicy with a narcissus or banana-like overtone.

Essential oils can be used with a diffuser, added to a bath during a skin care ritual, or added to an unscented lotion so they can be inhaled all day for lasting benefits. Try a drop or two of lavender oil on your pillow at night to help you sleep or put a drop or two of bergamot oil in your tea for a relaxing afternoon break. Or light an aromatherapy candle while you read or while preparing for bed.

Aromatherapy might not cure everything that ails you, but it can certainly enhance your self-care efforts and create a tranquil mood when you're feeling overwhelmed and agitated by the world.

Chapter 8
Creating Your Introvert Retreat

"I want my home to be that kind of place—a place of sustenance, a place of invitation, a place of welcome."

—Mary DeMuth

Introverts spend a lot of time at home, and our homes are sacred places—or at least they should be. This is where most of us go to rest, reenergize, and enjoy many of our solitary activities.

It's taken me years to figure out exactly what "feels right" related to the best style of home design and the interior and exterior decor to suit my personality.

When I was raising three children, we had a home with a big, open floor plan. I thought this was ideal at the time because we could all be together even in different rooms, and I could keep track of what the kids were doing. If they were in their bedrooms, they could easily yell downstairs if they needed me. Which they did. A lot.

I didn't realize how a big open floor plan like this with five people milling around the same spaces and yelling from one room to another could be such a drain. If I needed quiet and privacy, I had to go into my bedroom and lock the door. Even my office was doorless and available for people to easily interrupt me.

Now I'm an empty nester and there are just two of us (both introverts). My home is a peaceful haven even though I still have some open spaces. I also have some quiet and cozy spaces. The rooms are uncluttered, and the decor is minimalist and modern, which is a change from my typical design preferences. But what a positive change it has made on my psyche.

If you haven't paid much attention to how your environment affects you, then right now is a good time to start as part of your self-care plan. Think about how your home can foster and nurture your quiet and contemplative nature.

If you're a highly sensitive introvert, then it's even more important that your home is a respite because of your enhanced sensitivities to light, noise, smells, and the moods of those around you.

You can start this process by asking yourself a few questions.

- In what parts of my home do I feel the most comfortable and happy?
- What parts make me feel uncomfortable, drained, edgy, or unhappy?
- Are my bedroom and bathroom conducive to winding down for sleep rituals?
- Is the floor plan of my home suitable for my introverted nature?
- Do the decor and furnishings reflect my personality and work for my lifestyle?
- Are there smells, noises, and lighting that bother me in my home?
- Is my home cluttered, and, if so, does that agitate me?
- Can I find the privacy I need both indoors and outdoors at my home?

- Do I have an outdoor area that feels peaceful and makes me happy?

- Do I have a good space for intimate conversations?

Once you have the answers to these questions, you'll have a better idea of what you need to do to make your home more of a retreat that supports you mentally and physically. You might not be able to afford or have the time to make any major structural changes or buy new furniture, but there are things you can do easily to make your home more introvert-friendly.

Ged Rid of Clutter

As an introvert, I find tidying and organizing my stuff a complete bore. It seems like a task that pulls me away from what I really want to be doing —writing, reading, listening to music, hiking, or having intimate conversations. But I've found that clutter and disorganization is a huge drain for me. It saps my energy and makes me feel anxious.

I think clutter makes most people feel this way, although some are better at overlooking it than others. Whether you're consciously aware of it, clutter does have a negative impact on your psyche and mind.

In a 2011 study,* neuroscientists at Princeton University looked at people's task performance in an organized versus disorganized environment and found that physical clutter in your surroundings competes for your attention, decreasing your performance and increasing stress. Another study* revealed that the stress hormones of mothers spiked during the time they spent dealing with their belongings.

Like me, you might not like decluttering and find it a waste of time. If so, then hire someone who is good at it to work for a few hours. You can find inexpensive, personal organizers by searching online in your area. If you want to try it yourself, check out my book (with coauthor S. J. Scott), *10-Minute Declutter: The Stress-Free Habit for Simplifying Your Home.*

Decide on the room that needs the most attention or the area that you most want to declutter, so you can better enjoy the space. Then start with one small section at a time, working your way around the room. Let go of as much stuff as you can—things that you don't use, that take up space, or that don't make you happy. Letting go of draining physical stuff is as much a self-care activity as redecorating a room.

Marie Kondo, the author of the *New York Times* bestseller, *The Life-Changing Magic of Tidying Up*, suggests, "**To truly cherish the things that are important to you, you must first discard those that have outlived their purpose**. To get rid of what you no longer need is neither wasteful nor shameful" (bold text in original, page 61).

Make Your Bedroom and Bathroom a Zen Retreat

Many of the self-care strategies I present here take place in your bedroom or bathroom. But if these rooms are filled with clutter and dirty clothes or if the decor is drab or uninspiring, then your self-care won't feel as pleasurable.

Think about how it feels to walk into a luxurious, spa-like hotel room that just whispers, "relax." If you haven't been in one, you've certainly seen photos. By changing a few items in your bedroom and bathroom, you can create this feeling for yourself.

A fluffy comforter, new pillows, soft incandescent lighting, and some candles can change the entire feel of your bedroom. If you need some ideas, visit Pinterest and type in "spa bedroom ideas" or "minimalist bedroom ideas," and you'll find plenty of inspiration.

The same goes for your bathroom. A few changes, like painting dated cabinets, updating the mirror and light fixtures, and adding new towels and bath accessories can make a huge difference in how your bathroom feels.

Create Special Nooks

If you love to read, write, create, journal, or just sit and think, it's so much more inspiring to have the right space to do these things. Do you have a small room or space in your home that you can transform into a special nook for quiet creative or contemplative time?

If you need ideas, visit Pinterest again and type in "reading nook," "writing nook," "art spaces," "sacred spaces," "prayer room," or any other type of private space depending on what you want to use it for.

If you can afford it, consider getting an outdoor shed or tiny house that you can use as your own private studio or getaway. There's an entire movement around "she sheds" (the woman's version of man caves), but men can also enjoy these outdoor spaces.

You'll find tons of ideas for "she sheds" on Pinterest by searching online for that term. Guys, you can also find great ideas for outdoor spaces for your hobbies or creative pursuits by looking up "man sheds."

There are plenty of prefab shed options you can purchase and design to your specifications (check out the article* "Five Cool Prefab Backyard Sheds You Can Buy Right Now," which reviews several companies that build backyard sheds). If you're handy and like to build things, you can easily find "do-it-yourself" shed kits online or at Lowe's, Menards, and The Home Depot.

Create a Private Garden Area

If a shed or outdoor studio isn't in your budget, then consider a private garden area or patio that you can use as a retreat. You don't have to spend a lot of money to plant shrubs for privacy (or put up a screen) and flowers for beauty.

If it's in the budget, build or buy a small firepit for cozy evenings with a glass of wine or add a waterfall fountain for soothing background noise. Wind chimes are a nice addition too. I found some beautiful ideas on Pinterest by typing in "cozy garden sitting areas."

If a garden feels too overwhelming, consider putting up a porch swing, a hammock, or even a hanging daybed that can be made easily by a handyperson or carpenter. The article* "Thirty-Seven Smart DIY Hanging Bed Tutorials and Ideas to Do," has some fantastic ideas for the coziest hanging beds.

Liven Up Your Living Spaces

Other than your bedroom, bathroom, and cozy nook, where do you spend most of your time? In your family room, kitchen, or basement? Invest some time in making these spaces more inviting and soothing.

Add some fresh flowers and houseplants to bring the outdoors in. Sign up for Spotify or Pandora so you can have soothing or inspiring music playing at the push of a button. Choose some artwork (it doesn't have to be expensive) that speaks to you and reflects your style.

Rearrange furniture (or remove some of it) to better suit how you live. Paint a room, modernize your lampshades, and update a tired look with new pillows and throws. Find an inexpensive area rug (try IKEA, Target, West Elm, or CB2) to give a more modern and cohesive look.

If you love to cook and spend a lot of time in your kitchen, update your utensils and cookware. Get rid of old stuff that clutters your drawers and cabinets. Make your kitchen a space you look forward to spending time in rather than just the room where you make food.

Your environment plays such a big role in your motivation, peace of mind, and happiness. Having a home that you look forward to spending time in will ensure that you take better care of yourself physically and mentally. You might not be able to tackle all of these suggestions but pick one or two that you can easily accomplish by taking small actions every day.

Paying attention to your environment, body, and physical needs is an essential part of your self-care plan. But as you know, your body, mind, and emotions work together and affect one another.

Even when you are treating your body with TLC, you can't ignore your inner world and how you manage your time, thoughts, and emotions to feel balanced and mentally calm. Because you spend so much time in your inner world, it is even more essential that you understand how to take care of your mental and emotional health.

SECTION 2

MENTAL AND EMOTIONAL SELF-CARE

"You are beautiful because you let yourself feel, and that is a brave thing indeed."

—Shinji Moon

In her book, *Quiet*, Susan Cain notes that during the late 1940s, the provost of Harvard University suggested that the university should turn down applicants who are "the 'sensitive, neurotic' type and the 'intellectually over-stimulated.'" In 1950, Yale's president agreed, stating that the ideal Yale student should not be a "beetle-browed, highly specialized intellectual, but a well-rounded man" (page 28).

By the time students were matriculating into Harvard or Yale in the mid-1900s, the extrovert ideal was firmly established. Introversion was viewed as a handicap to personal and professional success, if not a full-blown mental disorder. Despite Jung's efforts to shed light on the introverted personality and even normalize it, Western culture has continued to stigmatize those who aren't gregarious "world dominators."

The Stigma of Introversion

As recently as 2010, the American Psychiatric Association (APA) was considering the inclusion of introversion as an indicator in psychopathology in its *Diagnostic and Statistical Manual of Mental Disorders* (*DSM-5*). The APA labeled introversion as a contributing factor in diagnosing certain personality disorders.

The main professional organization of psychiatrists in the United States, the largest psychiatric organization in the world, wanted to include introversion in its standard classification of mental disorders. After much outcry from introverts and many in the psychiatric community, the APA has removed "introversion" from the most recent version of the *DSM-5* but still hedges on giving introverts a clean bill of mental health.

In a 2012 article in Psychology Today,* Laurie Helgoe, clinical psychologist and author of *Introvert Power*, says:

> It's ironic that psychiatry—the profession that produced Carl Jung and liberated so many by enriching our understanding of personality—also has the power to reduce and pathologize those at one end of the personality spectrum. That is a sobering power, and one that needs many checks.

With all the stigma surrounding introversion, even from the mental health community, it's no wonder that introverts have complicated feelings about themselves and how they interact with the world.

If society didn't suggest we need to be more sociable, gregarious, and aggressive, most of us introverts would be perfectly fine with who we are, thank you very much. Living a quiet-ish life, having a handful of close friends, and preferring a good book over a loud shindig would feel perfectly normal.

When I was younger, I spent years forcing myself to stay out late with friends, engaging in small talk I had little interest in and could barely hear over loud music. I didn't want to be the boring party pooper, so I feigned enthusiasm I didn't feel. No one would have known that I was counting the minutes until it was reasonable to say, "I've got to go home now."

I remained in a public relations career that would have been perfect for an extrovert, but too often it wore me out and left me longing for something more meaningful. I pressed on because I assumed all jobs were meant to be stressful and exhausting.

An introverted friend who was a minister for over a decade didn't realize until recently he'd chosen a tortuous career for his personality type. He preached every Sunday in front of hundreds of people, followed by lots of handshaking and small talk once the service was over. He was so exhausted afterward that he'd spend the remainder of the weekend on the couch recovering.

For my friend and me, we didn't know we were doing ourselves a disservice by trying to fit in with the extrovert ideal. We wanted to be part of the group, viewed as sociable and confident. We felt that if we just kept working at it, pushing ourselves to adapt, it would get easier over time.

In some ways it did get easier, as anything does that you do repeatedly, but our basic personalities haven't changed. We now both feel comfortable in our introverted shoes, with enough extroversion to enjoy a satisfying professional and social life—but on our own terms and without worrying that others will judge us as antisocial or shy.

Often confused with shyness, introversion doesn't imply social awkwardness or anxiety. Most introverts don't choose to be alone because they are withdrawn or depressed. They choose to be alone (or with a small group) because they prefer quiet time to think and process. They enjoy more intimate conversations. They need to drown out the noise and stimulation of everyday life, so they can recharge their batteries.

Mental Health for Introverts

Unfortunately, the noise and stimulation around us aren't getting any less intense, and the demands for introverts to adapt or be pushed aside are as fierce as ever. Laurie Helgoe nails this dilemma in a *Psychology Today* article,* saying,

> As American life becomes increasingly competitive and aggressive, to say nothing of blindingly fast, the pressures to produce on demand, be a team player, and make snap decisions cut introverts off from their inner power source, leaving them stressed and depleted. Introverts today face one overarching challenge—not to feel like misfits in their own culture.

It's no wonder that introverts (more than extroverts) *do* deal with depression, anxiety, and sleeplessness. When you feel you don't fit in, can't compete fairly with extroverts, and are viewed as flawed, it can take a toll on your mental health.

Introverts also can be highly self-critical and perfectionistic. (Sound familiar?) Even when they perform to the best of their abilities, they often aren't satisfied with their efforts, leaving them mentally and physically exhausted. More than most, introverts tend to worry about what others think of them, causing additional anxiety and stress.

Both introverts and extroverts can become depressed, but it appears that there are far more depressed introverts than extroverts. A 2002 study* published in the *Journal of Psychiatric Research* found that introverts made up 74 percent of the depressed population.

This research seems to contradict the fact that introversion should not be pathologized. If most depressed people are introverts, it's not a far leap to assume introversion causes depression. Although introversion doesn't *cause* depression, there are plenty of reasons that introverts might be more *susceptible* to anxiety and depression.

- Given that our culture favors extroversion in everything from media messaging to hiring practices, introverts do face more challenges in their efforts to succeed and be valued. They are expected to adapt in ways that are not only unnatural but also depleting and stressful.

- Some (not all) introverts feel inadequate because of cultural stigmas and their own self-critical natures, making them question their worthiness and value in society. This can affect their ability to perform their best, further deflating their sense of confidence and self-esteem.

- Because introverts spend more time processing information, they might ruminate on negative thoughts and emotions, stirring up feelings of sadness and anxiety. As a result, they might withdraw from their social circles, compounding their negative feelings with a sense of isolation.

All these reasons create the perfect storm for mental health problems for someone who might otherwise be happy and satisfied with who they are and how they operate in the world.

Of course, these scenarios don't describe all introverts, and you might not see yourself in any of them. But even the most mentally healthy introverts should be aware of the propensity we have for pondering, fretting, and brooding. We need to pay attention to our moods and gauge our state of mind on a daily basis to become aware of our mental patterns.

Mindfully tending to your mental and emotional health is a pivotal part of your self-care plan. Understanding more about yourself and what it means to be an introvert should be the foundation of this plan.

This self-awareness allows you take precautions to protect your psyche from overstimulation, unproductive thinking, and over-scheduling. It also gives you the confidence to live authentically, true to your introverted needs and preferences, without feeling guilty or flawed.

Even if you feel completely self-assured about your introverted nature, you need to prioritize your mental and emotional care to thrive and perform optimally in your personal and professional life.

Let's talk about some of the ways you can practice self-care for your inner world so that you are centered, energized, and productive.

In Section 2, we'll go through these nine mental and emotional self-care strategies.

1) Practice mindfulness.

2) Spend time in nature.

3) Read for pleasure.

4) Explore creative outlets.

5) Protect your time.

6) Enforce digital breaks.

7) Treat mental health problems.

8) Find vitality and meaning.

9) Create emotional outlets and buffers.

Let's get started!

Chapter 9
Practice Mindfulness

*"In today's rush, we all think too much, seek too much, want
too much and forget about the joy of just being."*

—Eckhart Tolle

American psychologist and founder of the Insight Meditation Community of Washington, DC, Dr. Tara Brach, teaches that the only path to spiritual and emotional freedom is by awakening from the "trance of thinking."

What does she mean by the "trance of thinking"? Dr. Brach suggests that our incessant thoughts separate us from the only true reality—the present moment. Our thoughts also cause us profound suffering because we are so attached to them and believe everything we think.

But if we start to notice when our thoughts are not serving us, we discover that we have a choice. We can stay locked in our thoughts, careening from one anxiety to another, or we can return to the present moment where there is always peace. We don't have to allow our thoughts to control our experience of life. We don't even have to believe our own thoughts, especially the negative thoughts, which are so often grounded in untruth.

This choice is powerful and liberating for introverts who prefer the corridors of their minds to the bustling hallways of their work environments or the dizzying demands of social events. Without engaging this choice, introverts can easily become trapped in the trance of thinking. If we aren't careful, we can spin never-ending webs of thought that devolve into negativity, rumination, and worry.

Not that all thought is bad. Our proclivity for deep thinking and creative brainstorming is one of our greatest strengths. Our preference to think before speaking and acting, to ponder problems meticulously, and to process abstract thought, are what make introverts so unique and valuable. But it's *the type* of thought that counts.

As interesting and compelling as your inner world might be, there are times when you must return to the present moment for your own mental health. The more we are "in our heads," the more opportunity there is for obsessing and ruminating. That's where mindfulness practices come in as a potent opportunity for self-care.

Mindfulness means paying attention—being present in the here and now. Of course, this isn't something you can do 24/7, but you can adopt specific practices that allow you to escape the trance of thinking for a period of time. With practice, you will find you have more control over your thoughts than they have over you.

As I say in my book, *Peace of Mindfulness,*

> *Mindfulness is the intentional yet gentle effort to be present with experience in a nonjudgmental way. When you are mindful, you are right here, right now, with a conscious, purposeful awareness of the present moment. You're not dwelling in the past nor focused on the future—unless you are doing so with mindful intention. You are attentively immersed in the moment (page 5).*

The benefits of mindfulness practices are numerous and well-documented, not just for introverts but for anyone. You'll find that mindfulness improves your memory, reduces the tendency to ruminate and react, and helps you feel less stressed and agitated. It has also been shown to have a variety of physical health benefits. You can read more about the benefits of mindfulness in the post "Mindfulness Practice: Eight Powerful Benefits" on my blog.

Suffice it to say, practicing mindfulness is a habit everyone should adopt—but especially introverts. The question you might be asking now is, "How do I practice mindfulness?" There are many ways to become more mindful and wake up from the "trance of thinking." Let's go over some that you can include in your self-care plan.

Mindfulness Meditation

Mindfulness meditation is the Western, research-based version of Vipassana or insight meditation, a 2,500-year-old Buddhist practice. Today mindfulness meditation has no religious affiliation and is designed to help you develop the skill of mindfulness in daily life.

Practicing this meditation daily, for just fifteen to twenty minutes, will help you develop your mindfulness muscle and tame your "monkey mind," which tends to bounce around from one thought to another. Over time, you'll find it's much easier to be the witness to your thoughts and sensations. You'll experience a profound peace in the quiet of your mind and awaken to the joy in the present moment.

The process of mindfulness meditation is quite simple, but it's the consistent practice of it that takes commitment. If you view meditation as a way of taking care of yourself, the commitment to the practice will be easier.

Here are the basic steps for a mindful meditation practice as I outline in *Peace of Mindfulness*.

1) *Sit comfortably either in a chair or cross-legged on the floor with a cushion. Keep your spine erect and your hands resting gently in your lap. Don't recline as you might fall asleep. Erect posture will help you stay alert and awake.*

2) *Close your eyes, or keep them open with a downward focused gaze, then take a few deep cleansing breaths—maybe three or four.*

3) *Notice your body and the feeling of your body touching the chair or the floor. Be aware of your body in the space around you.*

4) *Gradually become aware of your breathing. Notice the air moving in and out through your nostrils and the rise and fall of your chest and abdomen. Allow your breaths to come naturally without forcing them.*

5) *Allow your attention to rest in the sensation of breathing, perhaps even mentally thinking the word "in" as you inhale and "out" as you exhale.*

6) *Every time your thoughts wander (which they will do a lot in the beginning), gently let them go and return to the sensation of breathing. Don't judge yourself or your intrusive thoughts. Just lead your mind back to focused attention on breathing.*

7) *As you focus on breathing, you'll likely notice other perceptions and sensations like sounds, physical discomfort,*

emotions, etc. Simply notice these as they arise in your awareness, and then gently return to the sensation of breathing.

8) *When you observe you've been lost in thought, detach yourself from the thoughts and view them as though you are an outside witness with no judgment or emotion. Label them by saying, "There are those intrusive thoughts again." Then again, return your attention to the breathing.*

Continue with these steps until you are increasingly just a witness of all sounds, sensations, emotions, and thoughts as they arise and pass away (pages 28–30).

You might consider writing down your experiences with meditation after every session to see how you improve over time and how meditation affects your thinking patterns. Ask yourself these questions.

- How intrusive were my thoughts during meditation?
- How successful was I at returning to my breathing?
- Did I judge myself for having intrusive thoughts?
- How successful was I at being a witness to my thoughts and sensations?
- How is meditation affecting my thoughts in general and my daily life?

Notice Your Thoughts

Throughout the day, your random thoughts can trigger anxiety, unhappiness, and anger and can keep your mind trapped in a cycle of longing and negativity. Rumination can become a bad habit for introverts that leads to suffering and undermines the quality of our lives.

When you apply mindfulness to your thoughts outside of meditation, you can change this cycle of suffering. By becoming the silent and dispassionate watcher of your thoughts, you understand how insubstantial and often misguided your thoughts are, freeing you from the emotional power they have over you.

Any easy way to begin noticing your thoughts is by using a physical reminder, like wearing a rubber band on your wrist. Seeing the rubber band will trigger you to stop and notice your negative thoughts.

- Just pretend to be an outside observer and look at your thoughts as you would notice clouds passing in the sky. Just notice, don't judge.

- Pay attention to how often you are focused on negativity, longing, or some distraction that pulls you away from the moment.

- Pay attention to how often your thoughts are in control and how your thought patterns affect your emotions and moods.

- Ask yourself, "Is this thought true? Is it based in fact or reality?" You don't have to believe all your thoughts. Most negative thoughts are based in assumption, magical thinking, worry, or regret about something that can't be changed.

- Gently redirect your thoughts to the task at hand or to a more positive, productive mindset.

Learning to take your thoughts less seriously is one of the best self-care activities an introvert can employ. We love thinking, pondering, and using our imaginations, but our active minds can turn on us. Mindfulness helps us filter the thoughts that don't serve us.

Mindfulness in Daily Life

The opportunity for mindfulness is in everything you do, in every task and seemingly unimportant activity of your day. When you align your attention and mental focus to whatever you are doing, you are truly living. You aren't regretting the past or longing for something in the future. You are here, now, experiencing the beauty and perfection of the moment.

For introverts, mindfulness can be just the escape you need when you feel overstimulated. Even in the most overwhelming moments, you can always return to your breathing, allowing it to anchor you to your body and the present moment.

In our hurried and hectic lives, when we race from one thing to another, it can be challenging to slow down enough to savor what you are doing in the moment you are doing it. But the benefits of slowing down allow you to have a more expansive acquaintance with even the most mundane tasks.

- When you make your morning coffee or tea, pay attention to each step. Notice the steam rising from your cup. Smell the aroma of the tea leaves or coffee beans. Savor each sip.

- When you wash the dishes, feel the water running over your hands. Notice the smoothness of the dish. Dry the dish thoroughly and tenderly.

- When you mow the lawn, notice the neat rows of mowed grass, the smell of the freshly cut lawn, and the way your body feels pushing the mower.

- When you are working, focus intently on the task at hand, giving it your full attention.

Bring attention and presence to whatever you are doing—from exercise to interactions with others—and you will discover a much more intense appreciation and joy in every element of your day. If the practice of daily mindfulness interests you, check out my book with coauthor Steve Scott, *10-Minute Mindfulness: 71 Habits for Living in the Present Moment.*

Chapter 10
Spend Time in Nature

"Look deep into nature, and then you will understand everything better."

—Albert Einstein

When I was a child, my mom enrolled me in Girl Scouts. I enjoyed the weekly meetings where my friends and I would make crafts, sing, and learn to cook Girl Scout Stew. But part of getting Girl Scout merit badges included going on overnight camping trips.

While some of the girls loved marching around in the woods, building campfires, and sleeping five to a tent on the cold, hard ground, me—not so much. I preferred to make forest fairylands with sticks and moss or play a quiet game with one or two friends. Most outdoor activities were not my cup of tea.

I did adore going to the beach as a child and have always felt a sense of peace and rejuvenation just being near the ocean. My idea of heaven is spending the day on a quiet beach with a good book, a beach chair, and a cooler filled with food and drink. As an adult, I've discovered a love for the mountains, having recently moved to Asheville, North Carolina, a city in the heart of the Blue Ridge Mountains.

As much as I love quiet time inside, I've learned that time in nature—whether it's hiking, running, biking, and other solitary or duo activities—can energize and revive me in a way that being indoors can't quite match.

I'm fortunate that I work from home and can take time to spend in nature whenever I wish. However, most people don't have that luxury. Between work, commuting, driving kids around, household chores, watching television, and spending time on digital devices, most of us spend the vast majority of our time cooped up.

According to the US Environmental Protection Agency* (EPA), Americans spend (on average) 93 percent of their life indoors or in a vehicle. That would have been nearly unheard of fifty years ago. If you live in a big city, you might spend little time at all in nature. For introverts and extroverts alike, this trend is taking a huge toll on our health and happiness.

There's plenty of science-backed evidence* to show why we need to spend more time outside and how beneficial time in nature is for our mental and emotional well-being.

Studies have shown that spending time in nature . . .

- Improves short-term memory.
- Restores mental energy.
- Produces feelings of awe.
- Reduces stress by lowering levels of the stress hormone, cortisol.
- Improves concentration.
- Boosts creative problem-solving.

- Eases symptoms of anxiety, depression, and other mood disorders.

- Improves sleep by resetting your circadian rhythm (during a weekend of camping).

In addition, being outside has many physical benefits, including reducing inflammation, improving vision, possible anticancer effects, boosting the immune system, and reducing the risk of early death.

For introverts, the mental health benefits are particularly notable. When you're overstimulated, overwhelmed, stressed-out, sleeping poorly, feeling blue, agitated, or lacking focus, getting outside for thirty minutes or more a day can make a huge difference in how you feel.

If you're an introvert who loathes the great outdoors and can't stand bugs, dirt, and extreme temperatures, you might need to challenge some of your limiting beliefs and find an outdoor "happy place" you can tolerate. You might find, as I did, that the benefits of being in nature outweigh the inconveniences.

Here are some ideas for enjoying nature in short and long ventures.

- Take a walk in your neighborhood, and be mindful of the smells, sounds, and sights around you.

- Plant a flower, butterfly, or vegetable garden.

- Go for a bike ride.

- Walk outside at night and gaze at the stars.

- Get interested in birdwatching.

- Find a beautiful waterfall or mountain hike near you.

- Take a weekend beach getaway (to a less-crowded beach).
- Take a weekend mountain getaway.
- Go river rafting or kayaking.
- Take up tennis or golf.
- Try an overnight camping trip.
- Get a dog (dog owners spend more time outside).
- Go on a picnic.
- Take an outdoor tai chi class.
- Visit a state or national park.
- Take up outdoor photography.
- Go fishing.
- Walk in the rain.
- Lie on your back and watch the clouds.
- Learn to identify different trees.
- Go horseback riding.
- Dine al fresco.
- Take your work or computer outside.
- Go on a guided outdoor adventure vacation.
- Get a hammock and read outside.

As an introvert, even an indoor-loving one, you can find refuge and peace in nature and outdoor activities. But you might want to steer clear of large outdoor events and festivals, team sports that require a lot of interaction, and guided group adventure travel where you can't escape to your own private spot.

Says introverted writer Nikki Hodgson, in an article* for *Adventure Journal,*

> I crave the silence of being alone in the woods, the way it falls around my shoulders. Being stuck in a group, even the best group, is difficult for me. I can't tune others out and my overactive mind processes and analyzes everything. I retreat because I am exhausted. I need a space without words, a space to close the door. A space that most expeditions and adventures don't easily allow.

You don't want to sour your experience of being in nature before you develop a self-care habit around it. If you spend most of your time indoors, start by adding a short walk to your daily routine or sit outside in the evening to watch the sunset. Consider practicing meditation outside for a few minutes a day.

Try to slowly increase the amount of time you spend outside, especially in the winter when you can be susceptible to seasonal affective disorder (SAD), a mood disorder characterized by depression that occurs during the colder, darker months.

Chapter 11
Read for Pleasure

"People say that life is the thing, but I prefer reading."
—Logan Pearsall Smith

When extroverts see an introvert staying home with a book on a Saturday night, they likely wonder why anyone would choose such self-deprivation when they could go out and socialize instead. For many extroverts, the idea of sitting alone for hours reading a book is worse than watching paint dry.

Of course, plenty of extroverts read books, but it's often for a specific purpose (that is, to learn a skill or acquire useful information) or to fill time when there's no one to talk to or nothing better to do. They often read the books that everyone is talking about—bestsellers and popular fiction that are fodder for good conversation and small talk at parties.

Introverts, on the other hand, pursue reading with a veracity that is near obsession. We read for the sheer pleasure of it, a pleasure that often outweighs the lure of any social opportunities.

Introverts can sit for hours with a book and view their time within the pages as time well-spent. Whether reading fiction or nonfiction, introverts read not just for pleasure and entertainment but with the purpose of gaining something meaningful and even transcendent from whatever we are reading.

With books, we can access the collective human experience without actually engaging in it. In fact, reading satisfies many of our needs for social interaction filtered through our own keen and hungry imaginations. We can live in any place or time, engage with various characters, and learn from creative and knowledgeable experts right from the comforts of home.

Writer Lauren Martin perfectly describes the intense pleasure of reading in an article for Elite Daily.*

Ever finished a book? I mean, truly finished one? Cover to cover. Closed the spine with that slow awakening that comes with reentering consciousness?

You take a breath, deep from the bottom of your lungs and sit there. Book in both hands, your head staring down at the cover, back page or wall in front of you.

You're grateful, thoughtful, pensive. You feel like a piece of you was just gained and lost. You've just experienced something deep, something intimate. (Maybe, erotic?) You just had an intense and somewhat transient metamorphosis.

Like falling in love with a stranger you will never see again, you ache with the yearning and sadness of an ended affair, but at the same time, feel satisfied. Full from the experience, the connection, the richness that comes after digesting another soul. You feel fed, if only for a little while.

Reading feeds our minds and hearts in a way that other activities can't muster. It is more than just an escape from the overwhelm of the outside world. Reading enlivens and enriches us. It sparks our imaginations and nourishes our souls.

As a self-care activity for introverts, reading has it's obvious pros—but it also has some potential cons. Reading is such a favorite pastime that many introverts can get lost in a book for hours. Most of us don't need any nudging to turn to a book when we feel overwhelmed or anxious.

Reading is a socially acceptable way to spend time alone to recharge and escape overstimulation, but it can also become a diversion that prevents us from other important areas of mental and physical self-care, like exercise, sleep, and social interaction.

Albert Einstein, an introvert, once remarked, "Reading, after a certain age, diverts the mind too much from its creative pursuits. Any man who reads too much and uses his own brain too little falls into lazy habits of thinking."

If you're an introvert who loves to read and can wrap yourself around a book for an entire weekend, your self-care might involve setting limits on the amount you read—lest you fall into lazy habits of thinking and doing.

The key is to find a balance between consuming and creating, between the inner world of ideas and imagination through books and the outer world of people, action, and things. Here are some strategies to make reading a healthy and beneficial self-care activity.

Manage Your Reading Time

Do you carry a book with you to lunch and seclude yourself to read while your office mates are socializing? Do you frequently spend hours a day curled up with an engaging novel, getting up only for food and bathroom breaks?

Slipping away with your book is relaxing and gratifying but be mindful of how often you do this. You might prefer the characters in your book to your coworkers but excluding yourself from these social moments could deprive you of opportunities to expand yourself professionally and build valuable relationships that help your career.

Spending hours immersed in your book might feel like a guilty pleasure, but you might be sacrificing essentials, like physical activity, time with the people you care about, or enjoyable experiences in nature.

Be proactive in deciding how much time you want to spend reading. If you grab your book automatically while others are around, consider engaging in a few minutes of conversation before you lock eyes with the pages. If you hunker down with your book on Friday evening, arrange time to spend with family and friends on Saturday.

Create a Reading Sanctuary

I like to read at night in bed, but there are cold or rainy days when I indulge in a few hours of recreational reading in the middle of the afternoon. I sit in a favorite chair that faces a big window looking out over the mountains. With a cup of tea, some soft music, and a cozy blanket, I'm completely content.

Do you have your own special "reading sanctuary"? If not, consider creating that perfect space with the right lighting, the most comfortable chair, and the best "feng shui" to make your reading time even more blissful. If you need some ideas, visit

Pinterest and type "reading nooks for adults" or "reading spots" in the search bar.

Make reading a special occasion of self-care rather than a convenient escape. Your reading time in this sanctuary can be a reward for finishing a project, completing your chores, or exercising.

Discuss the Books You Read

Expand your inner experience of reading by discussing the books you read with someone who enjoys hearing your opinions and thoughts. Maybe this is your spouse, your partner, or a friend who also loves to read.

If you're reading nonfiction, talk about the ideas and insights you're gaining from the book and how they affect you or how you can apply them. Describe the characters and the plot of your novel, and delve into any themes, metaphors, or symbols that spark your imagination. Talk about how books make you feel and what they evoke for you.

Articulating your experience with your book can strengthen your own creativity, help you formulate your thoughts, and build a closer connection with the person you are conversing with. As much as you savor the cocoon of your own inner adventures with a book, it can be rewarding to invite someone else into that world by talking about it.

Participate in a Book Club

Group events might not be your thing, but small group events might be, especially if the members of the group are like-minded people who also love to read. Joining a book club is another way to discuss books and share ideas and observations in a more meaningful and substantive way.

Introverts love deep and cerebral conversations, and you might discover a wonderful small tribe of people in a book club. The key is finding the right book club. You don't want to join a group who spends the first forty-five minutes socializing and only fifteen minutes discussing the book—or a group who tends to choose flighty romance novels or dime-novel mysteries.

The best way to ensure you join a group who shares your reading interests and your desire to focus more on the book than the small talk is to start your own group. If you manage the group, you'll have more control over the agenda and the genre. If this appeals to you, check out bookclubz.com* to help you manage and run your club and book selections.

But if you don't want to start a group of your own, there are plenty of places to find existing groups to join. Check out your local library and bookstores for book clubs in your area and contact the facilitators to get a feel for the types of books the group reads and the style of the meetings.

You can also find books clubs in your area by going to Book Club Meetups* or My-BookClub.com,* a free, online directory dedicated to pairing real-life book clubs with new members who can search by location, age, and genre. There are also online book clubs, like The Rumpus Book Club* or My-BookClub.com, that allow you to engage with other readers while staying in the quiet comfort of your home.

Listen to Audiobooks

Consider listening to audiobooks on occasion rather than always curling up with your ebook or print book. Most of us introverts prefer to read words rather than listen to them, but changing up the way you consume stories, ideas, and information every once in a while can be equally entertaining and enjoyable.

Audiobooks are perfect for road trips in the car when you can't be hands-free, or you want to share the book with your traveling sidekick. I love to listen to audiobooks when I'm on the treadmill, taking a long walk, or I just want to relax and listen to someone else tell me a story.

There are plenty of book purists out there who believe reading a book is somehow "better" than listening to one and that audiobooks are a cheater's way to learn or consume information. But for adult readers, research* shows that comprehension is the same for listening to and reading books, and that audiobooks actually have the advantage when it comes to clarity and intended meaning.

Chapter 12
Explore Creative Outlets

"There is an underlying, in-dwelling creative force infusing all of life—including ourselves."

—Julia Cameron

J.K. Rowling, the millionaire author of the Harry Potter books, is one of the world's most famous introverts. Writing books intrigued her as a child (she wrote her first book, *Rabbit*, at age six), but success as a writer eluded Rowling until she created the Harry Potter series.

Rowling shares* how she first came up with the idea for Harry Potter in 1990 while traveling alone on a train from Manchester to London.

> I had been writing almost continuously since the age of six but I had never been so excited about an idea before. To my immense frustration, I didn't have a pen that worked, and I was too shy to ask anybody if I could borrow one...," she writes.

> I did not have a functioning pen with me, but I do think that this was probably a good thing. I simply sat and thought, for four (delayed train) hours, while all the details bubbled up in my brain, and this scrawny, black-haired, bespectacled boy who didn't know he was a wizard became more and more real to me.

How was Rowling able to sit for hours pondering the future character of Harry Potter without being distracted by small talk with a seatmate or listening to music? How could she pass the time completely in her head, forging a story that would, in a few short years, change the trajectory of her life?

Because introverts, like Rowling, are able to focus for hours and hours, we can harness the motivation, attention, and mindfulness necessary for creative endeavors. This allows us to dive deep into the wellspring of our ideas and perceptions without feeling agitated or bored.

The most spectacularly creative people across a wide range of fields are introverts or introverted enough to be comfortable spending a lot of time alone. In fact, studies* suggest that solitude enhances creativity and innovation.

Says Susan Cain in her book, *Quiet,*

> *Some of our greatest ideas, art, and inventions—from the theory of evolution to van Gogh's sunflowers to the personal computer—came from quiet and cerebral people who knew how to tune in to their inner worlds and the treasures to be found there. Without introverts, the world would be devoid of:*
>
> - *the theory of gravity*
> - *the theory of relativity*
> - *Yeats's "The Second Coming"*
> - *Chopin's nocturnes*
> - *Proust's In Search of Lost Time*
> - *Peter Pan*
> - *Orwell's Nineteen Eighty-Four and Animal Farm*
> - *The Cat in the Hat*
> - *Charlie Brown*

- ○ *Schindler's List, E.T., and Close Encounters of the Third Kind*
- ○ *Google*
- ○ *Harry Potter (page 5)*

I'm not suggesting that extroverts lack creativity but that their creativity flows from a different source. It comes from being with other people, collaborating, and engaging with the world. Their brilliance is stimulated not as much from the inner world of thoughts and imagination as from the outer world of interaction and doing.

Introverts not only require quiet time alone for creative pursuits, but we also crave time to express ourselves creatively as part of our self-care process. We need uninhibited space to delve into our vivid inner worlds, to brainstorm, and to arrange ideas to produce something unique—whether it's a book or a new way to design a spreadsheet.

Says designer, art director, and digital storyteller Michael Champlin, in an article for the blog Introvert, Dear,*

> Creative space is about finding solace and silence in the external world, so that we may adequately listen to our own minds. This can mean different things to different people: writers may want time to read and jot down thoughts, painters time to paint, designers time to sketch, process, and brainstorm.
>
> Creativity is not a singular process, but rather an approach to every aspect of life, so it follows that not having time in our lives to express ourselves creatively—whether that's by painting watercolors or organizing our closets—can cause unrest in every other part of life.

As an introvert, you might already spend a lot of time in creative pursuits. Perhaps you have a job in a creative industry, or you strive to approach an otherwise unimaginative or analytical job with a creative and innovative mindset. These career-related endeavors can be deeply fulfilling, but they are still part of a job, often constrained by job performance anxiety and the demands of a client or supervisor who might not share your own creative vision.

It's when you are on your own time that you have unrestricted ability to cultivate your creativity for sheer pleasure and self-healing. While engaged in your creative endeavor of choice, focused and in the flow, you are recharging your batteries and tending to your creative longings.

When you are in the flow state, your brain secretes healthy doses of dopamine, serotonin, and norepinephrine, the pleasure-promoting chemicals. Creative pursuits infuse your life with a rush of good feelings and a depth and richness that is soul-satisfying.

If you are not creating on a regular basis, you're depriving yourself of an essential aspect of your nature. If you come home from work most days to lose yourself in social media, watch a movie, or even read a book, you are closing the door on so many opportunities for self-expression, innovation, and joy. What if J.K. Rowling had chosen to put on her headphones rather than spend her four-hour train ride quietly conjuring the magic of Harry Potter and Hogwarts School of Witchcraft and Wizardry?

Perhaps, like many introverts, you feel guilty for pursuing creative endeavors just for fun or relaxation. Maybe it feels indulgent or selfish, especially if you are a busy person with lots of personal and professional responsibilities. (And who isn't?) Please put guilt aside, my friend, because stifling your creative side comes with a price—like restlessness, apathy, and even depression.

If you need more convincing, studies* show that forty-five minutes of creative activity significantly reduces the stress hormone cortisol in the body, regardless of artistic experience or talent.

Let's explore how you can prioritize creative endeavors, no matter what your interests or expertise, to support your self-care as an introvert.

Carve Out the Time

You can easily devise dozens of reasons *not* to do something creative. You're tired. The dishes need washing. You don't know what creative project to work on. Most "right nows" don't seem like the best right now to delve into a project. It's easy to say, "I'll do that later when I feel like it and have more time."

That's why you have to make a date with creativity. Put it on your calendar and make it non-negotiable. Maybe you begin with a once-a-week date or an every-other-Saturday morning date. The key is to make a commitment to yourself that feels doable, and then stick to it.

Part of sticking to it requires that you plan ahead and set up your environment in a way that's conducive to immersing yourself in the project at hand. And that brings us to the next strategies.

Remove Distractions

Whether you are writing, drawing, or designing, you need a quiet and distraction-free space to plunge to the depths of your imagination. That means no phone (unless it's part of your project), no needy pets or people, and no other distractions that will interrupt your flow state.

Let the people in your home know to leave you alone for an hour or so. Close your door, clear your workspace, and get in the right frame of mind for your creative juices to flow.

Begin with a Short Meditation

One effective way to get in the right frame of mind is to begin the process with a short meditation. If you are carrying stress from work or trying to transition from family time to solitude, take a few minutes to calm your inner world and open the conduit for inspiration and ingenuity.

Close your eyes and take a few deep, cleansing breaths. Focus on your breathing for a few minutes, and then imagine a white light of inspiration filling your mind and energizing your entire body. Visualize the words flowing, the brush strokes effortlessly moving on the canvas, and the ideas spilling over in a torrent.

Prepare the Tools You Need in Advance

Don't waste your precious creative time trying to find the tools or materials you need. Prepare them in advance and have them accessible the moment you start your project. Let your tools be an invitation, calling you to put them to good use.

If you need time to clean or put away tools and materials after you're done, be sure you include that in your schedule.

Journal Your Ideas and Plans

If you aren't clear on exactly what you want to do with your project or where you want to go with it, use a journal to brainstorm, hash out ideas, and create your plan of action. Journaling is a creative undertaking on its own, and the process of using pen and paper to formulate ideas supports and enhances the creative process.

Just don't use journaling about your endeavor as a way to procrastinate on actually working on it. If you've set a limit on the amount of time you have to do something creative, then use that time for doing, and journal the night before as part of your preparation.

Suspend Self-Judgment and Perfectionism

This is hard for anyone pursuing something creative, and even harder for introverts who tend to dwell on their negative feelings and insecurities. Remember, this creative time is for self-care—it's not a competition or a statement about your talent or character.

Whatever it is you're doing creatively, allow yourself to be bad at it. Have no expectations about the quality of the final project except that you finish. In fact, avoid striving for perfection and rather strive for joy in the doing, *the process*. Just immerse yourself in the activity of being creative.

If you notice you're getting frustrated, self-critical, or angry while engaging in your creative project, then stop. Distract yourself with something else until you can return with joy and a positive frame of mind.

What If I Don't Know What Creative Project to Pursue?

When I turned 40 and was in the thick of raising children, I lamented the lack of creative time I had, given the demands of childrearing and running a household. It seemed any creative project I pursued would be interrupted by one of my three children or cut short by some other pressing responsibility, leaving me with an unfinished mess on my hands. This happened often enough for me to feel reticent about starting any creative activity.

A friend suggested I read the book, *The Artist's Way: A Spiritual Path to Higher Creativity* by Julia Cameron. Cameron teaches how to liberate and embrace your creativity, no matter how blocked, busy, or self-critical you might be. Reading this book inspired me to try pencil drawing, an activity that was easily interruptible without too much to clean up, put away, or leave strewn about.

I had no artistic training at all and no talent for it as far as I could discern. But as I began *the practice* of drawing, I became increasingly drawn to it (pun intended) and skilled at rendering what I was perceiving. I lost myself in the intricacies of lines and shades without the distraction of "trying" to draw a bird or a face.

To my great delight, my consistent efforts paid off in consistent improvement. But even if they hadn't, I was creating. I was doing something imaginative that was fun, uplifting, and relaxing.

If you're short on ideas and don't feel you have the natural talent for anything creative, don't let that stop you from activating your creative exploration. You might not be proficient at something, but you are creative. Proficiency is a byproduct of the practice of creativity. The practice is where you will reap the benefits.

Consider some of these ideas.

- cooking new recipes
- gardening
- landscaping
- drawing
- painting
- quilting
- metalworking
- learning an instrument
- organizing your closet
- interior design
- ceramic art
- digital design and coding
- genealogy
- cell phone app design
- coloring
- creating a video
- photography
- writing poems
- watercolor
- model building
- making a vision board
- arranging your Pinterest boards
- making a comic book
- needlepoint
- carpentry
- whittling
- brainstorming ideas for a problem or challenge
- learning origami
- creating a photo collage
- writing your manifesto
- practicing magic
- building a blog
- discovering new music
- planning an adventure
- car restoration
- starting a podcast
- arranging flowers
- making your own stationery
- designing your own board game

No matter what creative pursuit you choose, "just do it," as the Nike ad implores. Make it part of your regular self-care routine on a weekly, if not daily, basis. Immersed in the labyrinth of your own imagination, you'll discover a level of peace and inner renewal that will carry over into the more stimulating and depleting aspects of your day.

Chapter 13
Protect Your Time

"We must be master of our hours and days, not their servant."

—Adapted from William Frederick Book

"**Y**ou have to be good at multitasking, or you won't survive in the agency world." That's what my supervisor told me shortly after I left a corporate public relations job to join her fashion PR agency in New York. She was making clear to me her perceived distinction between the slower-paced corporate life and the hustle-bustle of agency work.

I needed to be adept at handling multiple clients and projects, quickly transitioning from one task to another, while managing a team of account executives and dealing with my supervisor's brusque and demanding temperament (although she didn't mention this part in her directive).

It was true—everything in my new job was faster, more aggressive, and more demanding of my time. Deliberative and slow thinking, taking time for pleasantries and manners, and focusing on one task at a time were not qualities that my supervisor appreciated or saw as valuable.

Although I worked hard to meet her demands and adapt to the agency culture, most days I dreaded going to work and often felt anxious and out-of-place. There were exciting aspects to the job, but the long hours, my supervisor's abrasive nature, and my own inner turmoil led to my resigning after a year from what was a coveted position.

In addition to being an introvert, I was also an introvert from the South, living and working in New York City, a place that was dizzying with noise, energy, and people living, working, and eating in close quarters. My time, space, and emotional energy were rarely my own.

In those early days of my career, I didn't understand myself well enough to seek out a job that supported my introverted traits. At work, I felt I had little control over how I spent my time or managed my energy. Even in my personal life, I felt I had to "get out there" and enjoy the intensity of living in New York and experiencing all the Big Apple had to offer.

Because of the environment I was in and my lack of self-awareness, I continued to swim against the tide, thinking that was my only option if I was going to be accepted as a valuable employee or a sociable friend.

You might be in a situation in your personal or professional life in which you feel the demands on your time and energy are too much. You might feel out-of-sync with the rhythms of your mental and emotional needs for downtime, quiet reflection, and less stimulation. Perhaps like I did, you feel trapped and unable to extricate yourself from circumstances that place burdensome demands on your psyche.

However, you do have more control over your time than you might believe. Certainly in your personal life, you can make some simple changes to protect your time. But even in your professional life, there are ways to set boundaries that help conform your situation to support your introverted needs.

Let's explore some self-care activities for managing your time and emotional energy.

Allow Enough Time

Are you one who presses the snooze button three times and finally gets out of bed with barely enough time to get dressed and out the door? Do you frequently run late or push deadlines to the last minute?

Most of us tend to underestimate the amount of time needed to get somewhere, finish a project, or complete a task. Or maybe we're so engaged in whatever we're doing that we don't allow enough transition time before the next thing on our plates.

Not allowing yourself enough time to do anything you need to do, whether it's to get to work by 9:00 a.m. or have the house clean before guests arrive, is stress-inducing and depleting. Introverts need time buffers that allow us to ease ourselves from one thing to the next. We need to feel we've had time to shut down one window of action before we open another.

It doesn't take much effort to give yourself this buffer. Even fifteen additional minutes can make the difference between feeling harried and overwhelmed and feeling calm and in control.

- Set your alarm a bit earlier in the morning and get up on the first ring. Give yourself time for a healthy breakfast and a short meditation before rushing out the door. If getting up earlier is difficult, start by setting the alarm just ten minutes earlier, and then add five minutes every few days until you can get up at your desired time.

- Add extra time to your estimate when planning a project or tackling a task. Calculate the longest amount of time you think it will take, and then add a substantial cushion to that time. Give yourself room to reflect, revise, and recalibrate once you finish.

- Think about possible roadblocks, pitfalls, disruptions, or challenges you might face when calculating your time needed for something. Consider your responses and alternatives in advance so you won't be caught off guard and pressed in the moment to find a solution.

- Prioritize process and flow over the speed at which you accomplish something. Unless you're up against a tight deadline, slow down as you work and try to savor what you're doing—whether it's cleaning the kitchen or writing a report. This goes back to being mindful in all of your endeavors.

By slowing down and giving yourself more than enough time to complete something, you are taking care of yourself and your innate needs to process and reflect. You're protecting yourself against the unnecessary stress and anxiety that rushing creates.

You might not accomplish as much in a day, but you'll feel more fulfilled by what you have accomplished and still maintain some reserves of energy. You are a quality over quantity person, so lean into that.

Simplify Your Schedule

When I had young children, I would create daily to-do lists that were impossibly long. I felt that the more I put on the list and crossed off, the more productive and valuable I was. I bought in to the popular notion at the time that women could and should "do everything and be everything," and my self-worth hinged on being a superwoman.

At the end of one particular day, I had checked everything off my long list and was finishing up the last load of laundry, feeling proud of myself for getting it all done. I folded the last item and looked in the laundry basket to ensure I hadn't missed anything when a pile of dirty clothes came tumbling down the laundry shoot and hit me on the head.

In that moment, feeling deflated and frustrated, I realized my work would never be "done." My list of chores would never be completed because taking care of a home and family isn't a one-and-done project. When this awareness literally hit me on the head, it inspired me to scale back my daily lists and try to focus on more time with my family and for me.

- If you feel overwhelmed or stressed by the demands on your time and energy, then recognize that simplifying your schedule won't be the end of the world—even if you disappoint other people or accomplish less in a given day.

- Begin by prioritizing what you want to accomplish each day. Depending on the amount of time each of these activities takes, shorten your to-do list to three or four items. Leave plenty of time for the activities that energize you and make you happy.

- If you've overcommitted yourself with volunteer or social activities, make some tough decisions about what you can give up. We often overcommit ourselves because we want to feel valued by others or because we have a hard time saying, "no."

- If you find yourself resisting or resenting something you've agreed to do, be honest and tell those involved that you are sorry, but you've overcommitted yourself. If necessary, help find a replacement.

- Be more discerning in the future about what you take on. Except in specific circumstances (that is, you want to support a friend or family member), don't allow obligation or guilt to be your reasons for overscheduling yourself.

- It might be harder to simplify your schedule at work, but you can try. Think about the meetings, interruptions, and time wasters that suck up valuable time and make your schedule feel tighter than it needs to be.

- Is it possible to eliminate some of these timesucks so you can focus more intently on the projects or tasks that really matter? Can you have a conversation with your manager about dropping these onerous tasks and explain how you need this time to be more thorough on the critical projects?

Leaving more white space between projects, allowing more time to complete tasks, and having fewer items on your daily schedule will give you breathing room and allow you to do what you do best—focus, create, imagine, analyze, and ponder.

These inner, solitary activities are the catalysts for your efforts in the outer world and allow you to create a reservoir of energy to fulfill your duties at home and at work.

Chapter 14
Enforce Digital Breaks

"We live in an age where there is a firehose of information, and there is no hierarchy of what is important and what is not."

—David Carr

The internet has been a boon for introverts. What once required phone calls, in-person meetings, networking, going to a library, attending a live concert, or visiting a shopping mall, can all be done behind a screen, all by yourself.

As an author, blogger, and course creator, I have the ideal career for an introvert. I work from home and can do everything I need to run my business from the convenience of my computer. Although I prefer socializing in person with my group of friends, I could rely on my smartphone and social media to interact with other people.

In fact, there's an entire generation of young people who primarily socialize this way, preferring to text, Snapchat, or Instagram their way to human connection. Their phones never leave their hands, and their eyes rarely leave the screen—even when they are in the physical presence of others.

As convenient and useful as it is, this technology has come with a cost, even for introverts. Intimacy is hard to achieve when your phone keeps beeping with alerts and notifications.

A constant, merciless distraction, our smartphones have come to replace the deep-felt, long conversations that introverts crave. For those of us who might have difficulty socializing, the internet gives us a further excuse to avoid reaching out to others or connecting face-to-face.

Why call your old high school buddy when you just saw his most recent update on Facebook? Why attend the conference if you can watch the video replay next week? Whether it makes us uncomfortable or not, human interaction is necessary for our mental health, and our digital devices get in the way of that. It's just too easy to get a quick dose of virtual interaction as a substitute for the real thing.

Not only do our digital devices affect our relationships, but they have a profound impact on our mental and physical health. In a study of students in ten countries, called "The World Unplugged,"* researchers reported that a majority of students experienced significant distress when they attempted to go without their devices for twenty-four hours.

Says Nancy Colier, author of *The Power of Off*, in an interview for the New York Times,* "Without open spaces and downtime, the nervous system never shuts down—it's in constant fight-or-flight mode. We're wired and tired all the time. Even computers reboot, but we're not doing it."

There's no question that our devices are disrupting sleep, according to many studies.* "Artificial light exposure between dusk and the time we go to bed at night suppresses release of the sleep-promoting hormone melatonin, enhances alertness and shifts circadian rhythms to a later hour—making it more difficult to fall asleep," says Charles Czeisler of Harvard Medical

School and Brigham and Women's Hospital in a National Sleep Foundation poll.*

Being continuously connected to your devices and constantly checking them has been linked with higher stress levels. "Many studies have observed that more time spent on social media is associated with an increased risk of loneliness and depression," according to an article in Medical News Today.* In addition, our computers and smartphones cause physical problems, including eyestrain, physical inactivity, spinal pressure, and neck strain.

Like so much else in life, moderation with our digital devices is key to a healthy relationship with technology. As an introvert, you might be more plugged in than others, given the solitary nature of the virtual world. But also as an introvert, you are all too aware of the drawbacks and potential problems associated with being connected 24/7.

For your mental and physical well-being, you need to unplug sometimes. Here are some thoughts on how you can do that.

Calculate How Much Time You Spend on Your Devices

From the moment you wake up tomorrow morning, be aware of when you are using your devices and for how long. In fact, when you turn on your phone or log in on your computer, make a note on the device about how much time you spent and what you were doing (working, texting, using social media, etc.). This will give you a true reflection of the time you spend in front of a screen every day. It will probably surprise you.

Determine Your Values about Devices and Other People

I don't think it's ever a good idea to have your face buried in your phone or computer when you are trying to communicate with someone else—especially someone you care about. But we all do this from time to time, whether it's waiting for a movie to begin, riding in the car with someone, or even in the middle of a conversation.

You can't really "be" with someone when you are distracted by your phone. Consider making a rule for yourself (and with your spouse, kids, and close friends) that devices are put away when you're together. They should never make an appearance at the family dinner table.

Consider a "no-bedroom" policy for your devices. This will not only help you sleep better, but also you might find you have more time to connect with your partner, have more sex, and indulge in some of the bedtime self-care activities I outlined earlier.

Choose Creativity or Physical Activity over Mindless Surfing

When we're bored, tired, or overstimulated, grabbing our phones and surfing the net or scrolling through social media is a quick and easy pacifier. It's also time wasted that could be spent on more fulfilling, enriching, or positive activities.

Try testing yourself with a twenty-four-hour freeze on mindless surfing. Put your phone or computer away and instead choose one of the self-care activities outlined in this book.

Take Regular Breaks If You Work on Your Computer

Sitting in a chair, staring at your computer all day for work is bad for your eyes, your posture, and your physical health. To protect your eyes, look up from the screen every few minutes and look into the distance for twenty seconds to allow your eyes a chance to refocus. After two hours of computer work, rest your eyes completely for ten or fifteen minutes.

Also, be sure you stand up and move around every hour or so if you sit a lot. After I've been working on my computer for a couple of hours, I'll get up to jump on my rebounder (a mini trampoline for exercise) or take a short walk. This helps clear my mind and re-energize me to get back to work.

Consider a Weekend or a Week-Long Digital Holiday

Could you be away from your devices for a weekend? How about a full week? It's sad to say that a digital holiday would be hard for most of us. I know I'd feel agitated and disconnected without my devices for a full week. But I also know it would a positive exercise.

The next time you plan a weekend getaway, try to leave your devices at home. It might be hard to travel without your phone, but if you're traveling with someone else, you can always make and receive emergency calls on his or her phone. Or leave your friends and family the number for the hotel or rental home you're staying in.

As much as we might believe we're missing something critical or that the world might end if we aren't plugged in, it just ain't so. In the gaping maw of emptiness created by your digital detox, you just might discover something amazing about yourself and the real world around you.

Chapter 15
Treat Mental Health Problems

"Promise me you'll always remember—you're braver than you believe, and stronger than you seem, and smarter than you think."

—Pooh's Grand Adventure: The Search for Christopher Robin

As I mentioned in the beginning of this section, introverts on a whole experience more mental health problems than extroverts. Our introversion doesn't cause us to have these problems, but it does make us more susceptible to them— especially when we don't take care of ourselves.

Taking care of ourselves often involves pushing back against cultural expectations, leaving a job or career that is ill-suited to our natures, and risking the appearance of being antisocial to recharge. It can take an enormous amount of energy to live authentically as an introvert. The pressure to conform can sometimes be as daunting as the energy it requires to give in and fake it.

Even for those of us who are in careers suited to our introverted personalities, who have supportive and appreciative family and friends, and who embrace our own introverted traits; stress, anxiety, and depression are still familiar companions. I have certainly dealt with all of these at different times in my adult life.

Like many introverts, when anxiety and depression first struck me, I was reticent to go to the doctor. My anxiety began as nightly insomnia and devolved into panic attacks and depression over the course of a few months. But I didn't believe I was depressed. I was sure if I could only get some sleep, I'd be better. I didn't realize my insomnia was a symptom of what was going on in my psyche.

For a variety of reasons, I waited a long time before I got the treatment I needed. I hated going to the doctor; I didn't want to admit I wasn't a superwoman, and; I thought I could diagnose and fix myself because I was obsessively reading about my symptoms and "at-home" treatments on the internet. If I'd sought the right treatment earlier, it would have taken a lot less time for me to feel better, be able to sleep, and resume my life.

When you're depressed or anxious, the last thing you want to do is get up off the couch, go to the doctor or therapist, or take medications that can make you lethargic or have uncomfortable side effects.

These mental illnesses cloud your judgment and kill your motivation to do anything except make it through the day. But depression and anxiety should not be taken lightly. They cause extreme mental (and physical) suffering, compromise your life and relationships, rob you of any joy, and can even lead to suicide if left untreated.

If you are experiencing the symptoms of anxiety or depression, you must seek treatment. This is one of the most important self-care practices you can undertake, no matter how resistant or unmotivated you feel.

Don't assume that the feelings will just "go away"—especially if you've had them for more than two weeks. Don't pretend that you have the knowledge or skill to diagnose or treat yourself. Don't allow so much time to go by without treatment that your symptoms become debilitating.

Let's go over how you can and must take action to address anxiety and depression before they get out of hand.

Know the Symptoms

We all have the occasional feelings of stress, agitation, sadness, or the blues. But when these feelings persist for more than a few weeks and begin to undermine your quality of life, it's time to act. Knowing the symptoms of these mental illnesses will help you act early to resolve them.

Anxiety Symptoms

- Panic, fear, and uneasiness
- Sleep problems
- Not being able to stay calm and still
- Cold, sweaty, numb, or tingling hands or feet
- Shortness of breath
- Heart palpitations
- Dry mouth
- Nausea
- Tense muscles
- Dizziness

—Web MD*

Depression Symptoms

- Trouble concentrating, remembering details, and making decisions
- Fatigue
- Feelings of guilt, worthlessness, and helplessness
- Pessimism and hopelessness
- Insomnia, early-morning wakefulness, or sleeping too much
- Irritability
- Restlessness
- Loss of interest in things once pleasurable, including sex
- Overeating or appetite loss
- Aches, pains, headaches, or cramps that won't go away
- Digestive problems that don't get better, even with treatment
- Persistent sad, anxious, or "empty" feelings
- Suicidal thoughts or attempts

—Web MD*

Go to Therapy

Studies* confirm that the best treatment for depression and anxiety disorders is a combination of psychotherapy and anti-depressant medication. The combination of both modalities has proven more beneficial than just one or the other.

If you are just treating your depression or anxiety with medication, or worse, you aren't treating it at all, you aren't affording yourself the full complement of treatment that can expedite your recovery.

One of the best forms of psychotherapy in treating anxiety and depression is cognitive-behavioral therapy* (CBT). CBT focuses on your moods and thoughts. By modifying your thought patterns, you can change your moods and behaviors. CBT relies on the idea that negative feelings and behaviors result from distorted perceptions or thoughts.

Some of these distorted thoughts might include the following.

- All-or-nothing thinking, where you can only see the bad or negative side of things.

- Disqualifying the positive things that happen to you and assuming they "don't count."

- Magnifying or minimizing the importance of an event.

- Having habitual negative reactions.

- Overgeneralizing and reaching broad conclusions.

- Taking things too personally

- Filtering out only the negative and focusing on it.

You and your CBT therapist work on identifying the negative thoughts and how you respond to them. Then you devise more constructive, positive ways to respond to stressors. You learn to control and change your negative thought patterns, practice positive self-talk, assess events and situations more realistically, and self-evaluate to respond more appropriately.

Go to the Doctor

The dreaded doctor—visiting him or her is not one of your favorite things to do, especially if you have to discuss symptoms that might make you feel embarrassed, weak, out-of-control, or shamed.

There is a stigma about mental illness, one that makes many sufferers (myself included) delay going to the doctor until the walls come crumbling down.

This stigma is fostered by a culture where feelings of vulnerability, sadness, and anxiety are considered weak and unacceptable. This is especially true for men, who are conditioned from youth that strong men don't cry. Even with increased media attention and awareness around mental health, studies* continue to show that a large swath of Americans still think that depression is the result of a weak will or a character deficit.

This stigma might add to your resistance to going to the doctor and discussing your symptoms—but go you must, especially if your symptoms are getting worse. Your doctor has encountered many patients dealing with mental illness, and he or she needs to rule out other possible physical causes for what's going on with you.

Your primary care physician can screen for depression or an anxiety disorder, but he or she might refer you to further evaluate your mood and determine whether or not medication is needed.

Consider Medication

When I first experienced a serious anxiety and depressive episode, I was adamant that I didn't want to take medication. I hated the idea of having to take antidepressants, and, of course, I had scoured the internet reading horror stories about them. So I tried herbal medications, exercise, and other alternative treatments—but to no avail.

By the time I finally met with a doctor, I knew I had to do something else. I'm so grateful for the care and education I received from this man who helped me find the right medication.

I'm not going to kid you—getting on and off antidepressants isn't easy for many people. There are side effects at the beginning that can be really bothersome. But after a few weeks, the symptoms generally fade, and you start to feel better. That's what happened for me and for thousands of others who take them.

They aren't magic pills, but antidepressants do help you find your footing and feel like yourself again. In combination with psychotherapy, they have proven to be an effective treatment. If you feel reticent to take medication, before you completely reject the idea, meet with a doctor or psychiatrist you trust, ask lots of questions, and educate yourself. Then you'll feel armed with enough information to make the right decision for you.

Accept Support from Family and Friends

When you feel anxious or depressed, you want to isolate yourself—more than you normally do. If you feel overstimulated around other people when you feel good, it might feel intolerable to be around others when you feel bad. But during this time, more than ever, you need to engage with the people you love and who care about you. Isolating yourself can make your depression and anxiety worse.

Those who are close to you can see that you aren't yourself and shutting them out of your life will only make them worry. It also adds more stress to your already distraught psyche to try to pretend everything is okay when it's not. I've found that being transparent and vulnerable with my friends and family gives me a sense of relief.

You might not feel up to chatting or going out but allow your loved ones to be in your presence, to prepare meals for you, handle chores, and take you to necessary appointments. Accept that there is nothing wrong with receiving help and support because you'd be there to help and support your loved ones if the shoe were on the other foot.

Treat Your Body Well

Many of the self-care activities outlined in this book are especially useful during the time you are recovering from a mental illness. Self-pampering activities (like taking long baths, getting a massage, and using aromatherapy) can be relaxing and soothing.

You might not feel like going for a run or going to the gym, but you can take short walks, practice yoga or tai chi, and do light aerobic activity at home. You can also allow plenty of time to sleep by going to bed earlier and waking up a bit later, if possible.

Support your treatment plan by eating a healthy diet with lots of water, fruits, vegetables, lean protein, and foods with omega-3 fatty acids. Avoid alcohol (a depressant), recreational drugs (which could interfere with medications and exacerbate symptoms), and sugar. If you're anxious, cut out caffeine.

Be Kind to Yourself

Introverts (especially highly sensitive introverts) tend to feel guilty. We feel bad when we offend or inconvenience others. We feel bad about ourselves when we fall short of our own expectations.

When I was in the throes of an anxious depression, I forced myself to get up and prepare breakfast for my family, get the kids to school, and follow my regular routine, even though every step was a struggle. I felt guilty for asking my husband to step in. I felt shame that my kids might perceive me as inattentive or distracted. I felt embarrassed that my friends saw me as less than fully capable.

Adding this extra layer of emotional pain is so unnecessary and counterproductive. As the Buddha is quoted to have said, "You, yourself, as much as anybody in the entire universe, deserve your love and affection."

This is the time to treat yourself with compassion and tender loving care—not guilt, shame, or recriminations. When the negative feelings about yourself and your mental health arise, try to step outside your inner turmoil to remember how deserving you are of tenderness.

Have Patience and Maintain Hope

Healing from a depression or anxiety disorder takes time. You will have plenty of bleak days when you wonder if you'll ever feel better. You might have unpleasant side effects from medication or experience painful times of self-awareness during therapy. You might take two steps forward, only to take three steps back.

Try to be patient and know that these are treatable illnesses, and you will get better. Try to maintain hope that you will soon have more good days than bad and that in time your life will return to normal or to a new normal that might be even better than before.

Chapter 16
Find Vitality and Meaning

"The meaning of life is whatever you ascribe it to be. Being alive is the meaning."

—Joseph Campbell

It wasn't until I hit midlife that I found vitality and meaning in my profession. Through my twenties and early thirties, I worked in a career promoting the goods and services of other people and organizations. The work was often stressful, sometimes a lot of fun, but rarely meaningful.

I stopped working for a few years to raise my young children (which was meaningful in a different way), but as they got older and needed me less, I craved more fulfillment outside my role as a mom and homemaker. I was deeply restless, feeling disconnected from myself and my purpose in life, but I had no idea what to do about it.

I tried to jumpstart my public relations consultancy, but my heart just wasn't in it. I had turned a corner in my inner growth and couldn't plod forward with a career that felt empty and purposeless. But what to do? I was forty-eight years old with no other employable skills—and I was fairly sure I didn't want to be "employed" anyway. I liked the freedom and flexibility of working for myself. It definitely suited my introverted preferences.

I knew I wanted something meaningful, something that supported and inspired other people. I was fascinated by psychology, personal development, emotional intelligence, and mental health. I was the friend who my friends came to when they wanted to talk about a problem or a challenge, and I loved that role. I was good at listening, analyzing situations, and helping them find solutions.

After much research, soul-searching, and trial and error, I made the decision to go back to school to get certified as a personal coach. When I finished coaching school and started to build a coaching practice, I created a blog to promote my services. As it turned out, the blog became the launching pad for a more fulfilling career than I could have imagined.

I wrote articles about the personal growth topics I was focused on with my coaching clients, and I rediscovered how much I love writing (something I hadn't done in a long time). I also discovered I could help a lot more people around the world by connecting with them through the internet.

That was the beginning of what has led to a full-time online business as a blogger, author, course creator, and teacher. I couldn't have scripted a better career for myself, but in truth, I helped in scripting it when I prioritized meaning and purpose for my work. As a result, everything else fell into place.

Not that I didn't have a big learning curve and a lot of hard work ahead of me—I did. But I loved what I was doing so much that the energy and discipline it took to start a business wasn't daunting but rather satisfying and purposeful.

Because introverts are inward turning, we tend to be more self-examined and self-aware. We know when our lives are misaligned with our values, integrity, and longing for meaning. That awareness can be a prickly thorn in our sides until we do something about it. Whether it's through our work, relationships, or any other aspect of our lives, meaning needs to be a driving force for our actions and choices.

Working just for the sake of making money or gaining prestige just doesn't cut the mustard for most of us. Having relationships only to fulfill our social needs doesn't seem worth the time and effort. Living a life that is rote and devoid of context and complexity isn't the kind of life worth pursuing.

We want something more. We crave something more. Finding ways to add more vitality and meaning to your life should be high on the list of self-care pursuits. Satisfying that longing and exploring the depths of your interests, creative inclinations, passions, relationships, and curiosity is a profound way to fill your reservoir of energy and well-being.

Here are some ways to ensure you're taking care of your need for meaning and purpose in your life.

Define What Meaning Is for You

For me, meaning is helping other people improve themselves and their lives. For you, it might mean inspiring others through art, educating young people, or creating a new software that makes life more convenient for everyone. It could be as simple as living in alignment with your values or being a caring friend or involved parent.

Think about what gives you a sense of purpose, meaning, and fulfillment. What feels important and valuable to you? How do

161

you want to leave your mark on the world—or just within your circle of family and friends?

Consider jobs, volunteer work, projects, or relationships in your past that you found meaningful, and ask yourself what made these things so worthwhile. Drill down to the specific actions or interactions that evoked a sense of meaning.

Pursue Personal Growth

Your tendency as an introvert to be self-examined has likely led you to many "aha" moments and periods of inner growth. But as part of your self-care, your goal should be to *mindfully cultivate* personal growth as a lifelong endeavor, a pursuit that is meaningful and fulfilling on its own.

This pursuit also will lead you to new opportunities, decisions, and mindsets that help you create a more intentional and fulfilling life.

Every day do something that satisfies your longing for meaning by enhancing your self-awareness and addressing the beliefs and behaviors that have held you back or caused problems in your life. Acknowledge that a meaningful life is possible only through radical self-honesty, personal responsibility, and the desire to grow beyond the limitations that keep us stuck.

Pursuing your personal growth can include these actions.

- Reading books by great thought leaders, psychologists, and other experts.

- Reading self-improvement and personal growth blogs.

- Attending seminars or workshops on personal growth topics.

- Taking online courses.

- Working with a personal coach or counselor.

- Listening to relevant podcasts.

- Talking with friends and family members who are growth-oriented.

I've included a list at the end of the book with some of my favorite resources for inspiration and personal growth. Reading, learning, and self-exploration are important first steps in your quest toward meaning, but this self-care work doesn't end here.

We have to do what many introverts are loathed to do—transform our thoughts into action. Without acting on your awareness, your search for meaning will become meaningless. This leads to the next steps in your self-care efforts for meaning.

Seek Your Passion and Purpose at Work

Think about this: you spend eight to ten hours a day at your job. That's more than half your waking hours in a day. If you don't like your job, you are spending half your day in a state of unhappiness or, at best, toleration. It's hard to find meaning when you spend so much time doing what feels meaningless, day in and day out.

It's easy for me to say, "Quit your job and go find something more meaningful." I know it's much more complicated than that. There are so many variables to consider and steps to take to begin the process, even if you know the kind of work you feel passionate about.

If you need help figuring out the steps, I teach an entire course (Path to Passion)* on the topic of finding your passion. And I have written about it many times on my blog. (Check out the article "How to Find Your Passion and Do the Work You Love,"* if you want to kickstart the process.)

Consider beginning the steps required for changing jobs, if you find your work lacking in meaning or not intrinsically motivating. You might not be able to change jobs next week, or next month, or even next year—but you can work toward figuring out how to get there in the next few years.

Imagine how much less stressed, overwhelmed, and apathetic you'd feel in a job that is a joy to perform. Imagine how much more energized, enthusiastic, and fulfilled you would be doing work you love that is meaningful.

Taking care of your introverted nature requires that you address this huge drain on your psyche and happiness. Addressing this one big issue could be the treatment for so many other challenges in your life.

Again, check out the list at the end of the book for resources on finding passionate and purposeful work and taking the steps to transition from your current job to a new one. As daunting and confusing as this process might feel now, it is a pursuit you will never regret, as it can be life-changing.

Help Other People

There is always meaning to be found in doing for others. Even as an introvert, there are plenty of ways you can help and support people and causes without doing something big and dramatic that requires too much of your emotional energy.

You might not be the one offering "free hugs" on the street corner or joining huge rallies. You might feel uncomfortable working in a soup kitchen or a homeless shelter. But you can certainly work behind-the-scenes for organizations doing marketing, fundraising, or writing.

You can be part of small volunteer groups or become a one-on-one mentor for a young person. You can work for a day on a Habitat for Humanity house, go read to an elderly person, or cuddle premature babies at a hospital.

You can find meaning in helping a neighbor, being available to a friend in need, or offering to help someone carry their groceries to the car. Small and discreet actions of service add up over time, especially when you become more intentional and proactive about your efforts. Need some other ideas? Consider these.

- Offer childcare for a busy mom.
- Become a pen pal with an elderly person.
- Send packages to armed forces service members overseas.
- Look for grant-writing opportunities.
- Walk dogs for an animal shelter.
- Plant or tend to a community garden.
- Write letters to your state and federal representatives about important issues.
- Clean up your local park.
- Participate in a charity run or walk.
- Create a blog about a cause that's important to you.
- Shelve books for your local library.

- Volunteer for administrative work for an organization or for a politician.

- Contact a nonprofit that intrigues you and offer your help behind-the-scenes.

It might not seem like self-care to help others, but if that caring adds to a reservoir of meaning in your life, you are also serving yourself. It feels good to help others and do something worthwhile for your community or for a greater cause. Decide how much time you can devote to service and be thoughtful in your choice of activities that give you a sense of vitality rather than deplete you.

Develop Your Emotional Intelligence

Emotional intelligence, or EQ, refers to the ability to recognize, understand, and manage our own emotions and recognize, understand, and influence the emotions of others. It is a critical component in your self-awareness and ability to relate well with others. A low EQ is not compatible with life meaning and fulfillment, as it's hard to find meaning when you're preoccupied with interpersonal conflict and inner turmoil.

Finding meaning and purpose requires that you are self-aware and also aware of how you affect others. It requires that you have empathy, integrity, open-mindedness, and a healthy (not oversized) ego.

Research* has proven that a stronger EQ translates to more general happiness, better mental and physical health, improved relationships, and a decrease in levels of cortisol (the stress hormone). For these reasons alone, the practice of strengthening your EQ should be in your daily self-care plan.

Someone with strong emotional intelligence possesses these abilities

- You think about emotions and how they affect you and others.

- You stop and think before speaking or acting.

- You resist being unduly influenced by your emotions and strive to control your thoughts.

- You view criticism (even unfounded) as an opportunity to learn.

- You show authenticity by saying what you mean, meaning what you say, and holding fast to your values and principles.

- You are empathetic, seeking to understand others' thoughts and feelings.

- You are able to sincerely praise and appreciate the success of other people.

- You offer constructive rather than negative feedback.

- You can apologize and take responsibility for your actions.

- You can let go of resentment and forgive.

- You honor your commitments.

- You are willing to help others.

- You remain open-minded about ideas and opinions.

- You are a good listener.

Emotional intelligence is a measurable component of who we are, just as IQ is. Studies show that although your level of EQ is relatively firm (based on personality and upbringing), it isn't unchangeable. If you are willing and desirous of improvement, you can change.

The best way to work on improving your EQ is by taking a test to see how emotionally intelligent you are now and where you need to improve. You can take a free, online version of the test at Emotional Intelligence Test.*

An excellent book on improving your EQ is *Emotional Intelligence: A 21-Day Step by Step Guide to Mastering Social Skills—Improve Your Relationships, and Boost Your EQ* by David Clark. Also, check out the article by Joshua Freedman on the blog, *Six Seconds*, called "How to Improve Emotional Intelligence: 10 Tips for Increasing Self-Awareness."* I list more resources for strengthening your EQ in the back of the book.

Develop Your Spiritual Life

Many people find profound meaning through their spiritual or religious beliefs and practices. If you are one of these people, and you've drifted away from your practices, then prioritizing them in your life might be an important part of your self-care.

Sometimes it can be difficult for introverts to follow a spiritual path because many spiritual traditions and religions promote the extrovert ideal. You're expected to be part of organized social events, outspoken about your faith, and active in the religious community.

In a culture where megachurches use theatrics, pageantry, and charismatic leadership to provide a "religious experience," introverts can find themselves on the outer edges of a faith community that feels alien and overwhelming.

Even so, introverts can still have a deep and rich spiritual life— whether that includes going to some kind of service or study group or examining life's profound questions in the quiet of your home. It's the *practice* of a spiritual life that is intriguing and enriching for us.

Says writer Alex Willging on the blog, Introvert, Dear,* "Why are introverts naturals at being spiritual? It's because we're quiet enough to hear the spirit, whether it's in the form of one god, many gods, the universe, or life itself." Our contemplative natures make us the perfect vessels for spiritual insights and communion with something greater than ourselves.

How can you develop your spiritual nature and engage in practices that are inspiring and transformative rather than taxing? Here are some ways you can care for yourself through your spiritual life.

- **Determine what your ideal practice is.**

Whether it's solitary devotional reading, practicing meditation, or being part of a small discussion group, figure out the practices that meet your spiritual goals without compromising your needs as an introvert. Pay attention to what inspires and uplifts you as you try different spiritual practices.

You don't have to join an organized faith group to have a satisfying spiritual life, but if that's meaningful for you, find one that doesn't demand too much from you in the way of socializing or proselytizing. There are many faiths that offer more contemplative variations of their doctrines that don't require you to be the life of the religious party.

- **Don't feel guilty about your spiritual choices.**

Unfortunately, guilt seems to be the lifeblood of too many religions. It's often used to get you to adhere to rules, donate money, and attend services dutifully, whether you want to or not.

I'm not trying to undermine anyone's religion or faith, but I know that guilt is rarely a positive motivator for a fulfilling spiritual life.

If you are practicing your faith in a way that feels uncomfortable or depleting because you feel guilty doing otherwise, please reconsider your practice. Remember, you're focusing on your spiritual practices for self-care—not self-flagellation. Only *you* know what fills your spiritual tank and connects with you in a way that feels meaningful and inspiring.

- **Find your own spiritual sanctuary for your practice.**

If you're not into organized religion or don't want to attend a regular service or meeting, create your own spiritual sanctuary. It might be a space in your home that you set aside for spiritual contemplation, a sanctuary garden in your backyard, or a spot in nature that feels majestic or peaceful.

Set aside time each day to spend in your spiritual cloister to read, contemplate, meditate, or pray—or whatever your spiritual practice might be.

- **Embrace your critical thinking skills and doubts.**

Introverts are deep thinkers and spend time pondering their beliefs and opinions. As a result, you might find yourself questioning some of your spiritual beliefs and resisting the idea that you must accept religious doctrine on faith alone.

Employing your critical thinking skills and having doubts are part of who you are and an essential aspect of your spiritual growth. It's also important that there are those in a faith community, often the deep thinkers and observers, who call out hypocrisy and point out weaknesses in ideology.

If you're an agnostic or an atheist, then critical thinking can lead you to your own form of enlightenment and a secular "spiritual" experience—whether it's through learning, time in nature, appreciating art and music, or some other transportive activity.

- **Practice faith through your actions.**

You might not be one to publicly express your faith or join an active religious community, but you can communicate your beliefs through your actions. You can reveal your beliefs, whether driven by faith or personal values, in the way you treat other people, through acts of service, and in how you reflect your integrity.

Chapter 17
Create Emotional Outlets and Buffers

"Because I rant not, neither rave of what I feel, can you be so
shallow as to dream that I feel nothing?"

—R. D. Blackmore

In 1989, Jerome Kagan, a professor of psychology at the Laboratory for Child Development at Harvard, began a longitudinal study that has linked introversion to reactions of babies in infancy. Four-month-old babies were presented with stimuli, like new sounds, faces, and objects. The babies who reacted strenuously to the new stimuli by crying and thrashing their limbs about were defined as "high reactive."

These more emotional babies were found to have overactive amygdalae—the part of the brain that triggers the adrenalin response to danger. As a result, the high reactive infants were easily overstimulated. Dr. Kagan continued to track the babies as they grew, and they became more quiet, careful children and teenagers.

Years later, another psychologist, Dr. Elaine Aron, drew on Kagan's study and other experiments on the tendency of introverts to be more sensitive to sensory, social, and emotional stimulation.

Through her research, she coined the term "highly sensitive" to explain an innate (and perfectly normal) trait held by 15 to 20 percent of the population. Of these highly sensitive people (HSP), 70 percent are introverts. Though not all introverts are HSPs, most HSPs are introverts. Maybe you're one of them.

Have you frequently heard from friends and family that you're too sensitive or thin-skinned? Do you feel overwhelmed by loud noises, bright lights, and new environments? Can you easily intuit and even feel what those around you are feeling? If so, you could be a highly sensitive introvert. If you want to know for sure, take Dr. Aron's short self-test,* and learn some of the specific behaviors and reactions of HSPs.

Dr. Aron has defined four core qualities of HSPs—(1) depth of processing and creativity, (2) being overstimulated easily, (3) being more sensitive to subtle stimuli, and (4) being emotionally reactive.

We've discussed how the first three qualities are common traits for many introverts and how to build self-care activities around these. However, if you are a highly sensitive introvert who is *emotionally reactive,* you might have some unique self-care needs that less-sensitive types don't require.

The HSP quality of emotional reactivity includes behaviors such as these.

- Reacting strongly to feedback, both positive and negative.
- Crying easily.
- Showing considerable empathy for others.
- Worrying more about others' reactions to negative events.
- Offering more positive feedback to others.
- Becoming angry, curious, sad, anxious, or joyful sooner than others.

Possessing a more emotional nature certainly has many upsides. Being in touch with your inner nature, showing empathy and concern for others, and feeling things deeply are profoundly rewarding. However, the depth of your emotions can be so intense that they are debilitating at times.

As I remind readers, in my book *Finely-Tuned: How to Thrive as a Highly Sensitive Person or Empath,*

> The characteristics of the HSP trait alone can set us up for emotional difficulties if we aren't mindful. We feel everything more intensely, and that includes the negative emotions that create stress, anxiety, and depression.
>
> We are more motivated to think deeply about things by our strong feelings of curiosity, fear, joy, and anger. It's hard for us to just let things go, so we ruminate about them for a long, long time, even when we want to quiet our minds and find peace (page 39).

A highly sensitive person feels the pain of other people and tends to worry in general about the sadness and suffering in the world. The emotional overload of taking on the pain of others is exhausting and can lead to mental health problems if it isn't balanced with enough emotional self-care.

Whether you are a highly sensitive introvert or an introvert with the emotional highs and lows that are part of being human, it's important to recognize when your emotional circuits have been blown and how to take care of yourself as you recover.

Here are some self-care strategies to create emotional outlets and buffers so you aren't depleted by your own feelings.

Learn about Your Highly Sensitive Nature

Do you have an inkling that you're a highly sensitive person? If so, take the time to learn more about this trait and how it affects you. Read Elaine Aron's book, *The Highly Sensitive Person: How to Thrive When the World Overwhelms You* and my book, *Finely-Tuned: How to Thrive as a Highly Sensitive Person or Empath.* There are also many other excellent books on the topic.

Once you know more about this trait and confirm you are an HSP, talk to your friends and family about it. Educate them on the HSP traits and how they are perfectly normal and positive. If necessary, ask them to stop referring to you as "too sensitive" and to respect any other emotional boundaries that you need to set.

Accept Your Feelings

If you've beat yourself up in the past about being too emotional or sensitive, recognize that there is nothing wrong with you. The more you learn about HSPs, you'll see that high sensitivity is a gift and should be celebrated. High sensitivity is an evolutionary trait that has benefited societies for thousands of years. As I mention in *Finely-Tuned,*

> Highly sensitive people are valuable and important to their communities and to the world at large. Because of your strong intuition and ability to sense what others don't, you are often the first line of defense (or offense) in helping those around you. You are the shamans, the mediators, the counselors, the physicians, and the healers that all societies for thousands of years have required for their survival (page 17).

You might not be in the majority as an introverted HSP, but you are no less "normal" than an extroverted person who lets everything roll off his or her back. Train yourself to have a new mindset if you've been trying to hide or reject your sensitivities.

This is especially important for HSP men who have been programmed to stuff their feelings and maintain a cultural standard of masculinity and strength.

Learn to Manage Guilt

According to Susan Cain, in her book, *Quiet*, "many introverts are prone from earliest childhood to strong guilt feelings" (page 234) and can feel an unnecessary amount of guilt, even in situations when they aren't guilty.

Guilt can serve as a motivator for positive change if you've done something wrong. Research has shown that people prone to guilt work harder, perform better at work, have more empathy, and are less prone to lie and cheat.

But sensitive introverts can allow guilt to fester long after we've rectified a situation. We even feel guilty when someone else is upset or angry, thinking their reactions must be our fault.

If you recognize this tendency in yourself, part of your self-care is having awareness about your extra sensitivity to "messing up" and the tendency for self-criticism. Self-criticism leads to less motivation and self-control while forgiving yourself has proven to increase personal accountability. Forgiveness beats unhealthy guilt every time.

Work on embracing that it's normal to make mistakes, hurt someone's feelings, or say the wrong thing, especially if you show healthy and appropriate remorse. How do you know what's healthy and appropriate?

Look at the intensity, duration, and consequences of your guilt related to the "bad deed." Would you punish someone you care about with the same amount of guilt for this action? Don't magnify an offense, as it will only make you feel guiltier.

You don't have to accept the emotional burden of another person's negative reactions and feel guilty because he or she isn't happy. If you are sensitive enough to notice even subtle mood changes in those around you, it's easy to extrapolate that you must be at fault or that you are responsible for "fixing" them.

Practice allowing others to have their emotions without assuming you need to say or do anything. Remember, it likely has nothing to do with you.

If you find yourself struggling with guilty feelings, remind yourself that feeling bad about yourself doesn't mean that you *are* bad. To be a good person, you don't need to be good all the time. Nor do you need to be responsible for the happiness and well-being of others.

Delay Responding to Negativity

Being around people who are critical, negative, or unkind can take a huge toll on your psyche. You might tend to internalize this negativity, dwell on it, and allow it to infect your state of mind. You might be inclined to react right away to fix the situation before you have time to process how you should respond.

Practice waiting a day before you respond to criticism or other negative remarks. Use your judgment (rather than emotions) to discern if the criticism has merit and if you can learn from it.

Try not to react with defensiveness or a knee-jerk apology right away. Give yourself time to think about the situation when you feel less reactive and can discern the best response.

Listen to Your Intuition

As one who is highly sensitive to everything going on around you, you might have little psychic space left for other things. You're devoting most of your energy to processing your emotions and experiences and trying to stay centered.

This doesn't leave much space in your head to listen to your intuition, which can often be subtle and require a clear mind. As sensitive as you are to your external world, you need to be more sensitive to your own internal world and what it's trying to communicate. This is a vital part of your emotional self-care.

Intuition is a well-researched phenomenon revealing that our brains have an amazing ability to pick up on patterns and respond to them in a nanosecond in the form of intuitive insights.

Paying attention to your intuition reduces stress, boosts creativity, makes you aware of potential danger, supports decision-making, and makes you more confident in your own judgment and wisdom.

You can make listening to your intuition part of your self-care with these actions.

- Meditating to calm and clear your mind to make room for intuition.

- Paying attention to your dreams, which are often symbolic and offer deeper messages.

- Running or jogging outside, which clears your head and can lead to "aha" insights.

- Taking a shower where the quiet space, warm water, and small enclosure lends itself to tapping into your intuition.

- Noticing sudden mood changes and asking yourself why your emotions have shifted.

- Noticing your body's reactions, which tells you through pain and disease that something is wrong or that you need to make a change.

- Taking a sabbatical or an extended break from your daily life and work, where you are completely disconnected from technology, distractions, and responsibilities.

- Thinking back over past hunches or moments of insight you've had that you didn't act on to see how your intuition was spot-on.

- Asking yourself a question about a problem or decision and listening quietly for the answer.

- Envisioning a conversation with a wise mentor or counselor, asking your questions, and listening to what this person has to say.

- Giving instructions to your subconscious mind before you go to bed at night to come up with the answers or solutions while you sleep.

- Trying to anticipate outcomes (of movies, conversations with friends, sports games, etc.) to tune into the mental patterns and connections that lead to the most obvious or natural result.

- Carrying a small notebook or using a phone app to make notes about your hunches and sudden bursts of ideas.

Practice Self-Acceptance

Everyone needs to practice self-acceptance, but as an introvert (and especially a highly sensitive one), you might be more prone to self-criticism and even disliking aspects of your personality because they aren't mainstream.

Underlying most of the emotional challenges we face, from depression to relationship problems, is the struggle for self-acceptance and self-love. Having a strong sense of self-worth allows you to accept yourself as you are and appreciate what you offer to the world. It is essential to being a fully actualized individual.

I could write an entire book on self-acceptance, why it's so important, and how to develop it. In fact, you might consider reading some books that I include in the resources at the end of this book on the topic. For now, here are a few daily self-care activities to consider if you're having trouble with self-acceptance.

- Start paying attention to the nature of your thoughts and how often you think negative things about yourself. This awareness will help you disengage from the thoughts, if only for a few minutes.

- Begin to filter your thoughts by applying the light of reality to them. Ask yourself, "Is my thought really the truth? Is it the entire truth or just my perception of the truth?"

- Envision yourself as your own best friend and think or speak only the words that you would say to your best friend in times of self-doubt.

- Set aside time to learn more about yourself—your personality, aptitudes, interests, etc. Take assessments, workshops, courses, and read books and blogs. See yourself as an interesting, multifaceted package to open and explore.

- Put yourself in situations and environments more often where you feel successful, confident, accepted, and happy.

- Find supportive friends who are easy to be around, caring, fun, and happy. Let go of people who put you down, try to manipulate you, or treat you poorly. Go online to find Meetup.com groups of introverts and highly sensitive people if you need help finding the right people.

- Practice realistic optimism about the parts of you that you don't like. Recognize that improvement is possible and working on an improvement goal will make you feel better about yourself.

- Practice loving acceptance of those things about yourself that you cannot change. There are really only two options— you can forever struggle against those unchangeable things, or you can grow beyond them and choose the path of self-acceptance. If you choose the latter, give yourself permission to stop focusing on your flaws.

- Develop a daily gratitude practice, so you can focus on the positive parts of yourself and your life.

Own a Pet

Introverts love animals—sometimes more than they love people. While our human companions can overwhelm or drain us, our animals tend to do the opposite—calm and replenish us. Animals provide unconditional love and affection, asking for little in return except for food and a little love and affection given back to them.

Pets can be the purr-fect (sorry, had to) buffer against the emotional turbulence that you encounter as an introvert, particularly a highly sensitive one. If a pet is right for you and your lifestyle, it can be a gratifying and delightful part of your self-care.

Research shows that our furry friends not only give us companionship and make us happy, but they also help relieve anxiety, stress, depression, and loneliness. According to a study* led by D. Helen Brooks from the University of Manchester in the United Kingdom, having a pet provides a deep sense of "ontological security," which is the feeling of stability, continuity, and meaning in one's life.

It probably won't surprise you that people who love cats are more likely to be more introverted, open-minded, and nonconformist, according to recent studies.* Dog people tend to be more extroverted and sociable, but some dog breeds can be loving, quiet companions that are perfect for introverts. If you are considering a dog, you might find this article, "What Dog Breed Should You Get Based on Your Personality Type?"* to be helpful and interesting.

Whatever kind of pet you get, try to pick an animal that suits not only your personality but also your schedule, living space, and willingness to care for it. You need to be able to afford food, grooming, vet bills, pet supplies, and pet care when you travel.

Try not to buy a pet on impulse (something introverts don't often do) but take the time to carefully consider if this is a good time to bring a pet into your world. If so, you might just find the perfect companion that sits in your lap or at your feet and quietly keeps you company.

Keep a Journal

Journaling has myriad science-backed benefits for introverts, such as enhancing creativity, reducing stress, and helping you process and heal your thoughts and feelings.

A journal is also a permanent record of your life journey that you can look back on over the years to see how you have changed and evolved. This helps you become more self-aware, compassionate, and intentional with your choices and actions.

Also, the daily act of journaling has one other hugely compelling benefit—it is an excellent mindfulness practice. When you write in your journal, your mind must be fully engaged with your writing. It forces your brain to slow down to better organize your thoughts and consider the big picture.

In the flow of journaling, past regrets and future worries lose their edge. You, your mind, and your pen and paper become one in the present moment. This state of mindful flow will occur regardless of the topic you are journaling about, as long as you are engaged in the process and find it enjoyable or cathartic.

There are many types of journaling that are worthwhile self-care exercises. You might consider journaling about one or more of these topics.

- Gratitude
- Daily moods
- Affirmations
- Answer a question or prompt
- Favorite quotes
- Stream of consciousness
- Your daily activities
- Dreams
- Meditation
- Prayer
- Travel
- Good memories
- Your children
- Your relationship
- The books you read
- Personal growth
- Goals and dreams
- Gardening or nature
- Creativity or art
- Planning and productivity
- One sentence a day or bullet journal

If you are new to journaling, you might want to start with a sentence a day or bullet journal to begin the habit of journaling. If you have an artistic bent, get a package of colorful pens for creative doodling in your journal. You might also try a journal with prompts rather than freestyle writing to help you stay focused.

As journaling becomes part of your daily self-care, you can expand your practice to suit your goals and needs. You might want to write more, doodle more, just use prompts, mind map—or a combination of journaling ideas. Check out some ideas on Pinterest by typing "how to journal" or "creative journaling ideas" in the search bar.

Do What Makes You Happy

This is a fairly obvious self-care directive—do what makes you happy rather than what makes you unhappy. But sometimes the most obvious actions are the hardest to take. Doing what makes us happy might not be socially acceptable, pay us a living wage, or be good for us in the long term. Maybe doing what makes us happy is guilt-inducing or feels selfish.

However, when you are feeling emotionally spent or overwhelmed, doing small things that make you happy can bring you back to center and provide the comfort and security you need to regain your equilibrium, so you can function optimally.

If you've had a stressful, intense day at work, perhaps going to your workout isn't the best choice. Maybe going home and curling up with your book is exactly what you need. If you feel overwhelmed by your friend's bad mood, and it's affecting your mood, maybe you need to go take a solo walk in the park.

When your emotions get the best of you, ask yourself, "What would make me happy right now?" If being happy isn't possible in the moment, then ask, "What would relieve some of this emotional intensity right now?" Create a list in advance of "happy things" you can do during these times, so you don't have to think too hard in the moment. You might find some ideas in the self-care activities listed throughout this book.

Over time, consider making some of the bigger changes in your life that will improve your happiness like one of the following.

- Changing jobs to something you love to do.
- Letting go of a draining relationship.
- Pursuing a long-held dream or goal.
- Moving to a city that is more aligned with your values and interests.
- Taking better care of your health and fitness.
- Saving money for travel, education, or hobbies.

There are many other emotional outlets and buffers that we've covered in previous chapters, including exercise, creative endeavors, meditation, spending time in nature, spiritual practice, and practicing soothing rituals for your body. Virtually all of these self-care activities can improve your mental well-being and serve as buffers against negative and debilitating emotions.

I've found that aerobic exercise helps to dissipate anxiety. When I feel blue, talking and laughing with a friend is the best cure. If I feel overwhelmed and stressed, taking a walk in nature is my go-to medicine. Through trial and error and practice, you'll find what works best for you in helping you regain emotional equilibrium when you're feeling off.

Conclusion

"In a gentle way, you can shake the world."
—Mahatma Gandhi

I hope the strategies I've outlined in this book have proven inspiring and useful for you. My work is done here, but yours is just beginning as you act to prioritize self-care in your daily life. I sincerely hope you won't just put this book aside without using the material to make positive changes in your life.

You might feel a bit overwhelmed by all the ideas I've presented, but your goal isn't to check everything off the list. It's to find what works for you, your lifestyle, and your particular needs as an introvert.

Pick a couple of strategies that you can easily add to your daily routine. Try them out for a few weeks and see if they help you feel more centered, balanced, and happy. Also, consider acting on some of the more time-consuming and dramatic life changes, like changing jobs or moving to a new city, if you find you are suffering as a result of being in the wrong place for your personality.

It takes time to implement these big changes but doing so can mean the difference between feeling trapped in an overwhelming, depleting situation or living more in alignment with who you are. The time it takes is nothing compared to the positive effects the change will have on your life.

In my research, I reached out to my introverted blog readers and social media followers to get their feedback and input on this book and the topic. Most people were enthusiastic, but a few responded defensively, wondering in essence, "Why do you think introverts need special treatment? There's nothing wrong with us!"

That is absolutely true—there is nothing wrong with you. Introversion is a normal personality trait held by a large percentage of the population. In fact, several studies exist to support that introverts are gifted. A study* by the Gifted Development Center found that about 60 percent of gifted children are introverted (compared with 30 percent of the general population) and 75 percent of highly gifted children are introverts.

I have mentioned throughout this book the unique, creative, powerful qualities introverts possess that make them so valuable as spouses, partners, friends, parents, children, employees, managers, and members of society. Introverts should feel proud and be confident in who they are.

I've also made you a little more aware of the reasons why self-care is so critical for your personality type—which does come with some unique challenges. It is these challenges in particular that call you to lift your head out of your book, up from the art table, or over the computer to pay attention and do something proactive so you can thrive.

As a reminder, here are some of the challenges introverts can face as a result of being introverted.

- Introverts are more susceptible to chronic illness and infection than their extroverted friends.

- Introverts tend to go to the doctor less frequently than extroverts and can receive substandard healthcare compared to extroverts.

- Introverts tend to avoid group fitness programs.

- Introverts get more overwhelmed and drained in social settings.

- Introverts tend to experience a higher degree of stress, anxiety, and depression than extroverts.

- Introverts have a propensity for sleep disorders.

- Introverts have a risk of isolating themselves too much.

- Introverts can be prone to sitting too much or being more sedentary than extroverts.

- Introverts might have more food sensitivities or values-based food restrictions.

- Introverts need quiet spaces for recharging, creativity, and rest.

- Introverts need to protect their time and energy more than extroverts.

- Introverts need creative outlets to feel fulfilled.

- Introverts crave meaning in their work and lives.

- Introverts tend to be self-critical and feel unhealthy guilt.

- Highly sensitive introverts are more reactive to external stimuli (light, noises, smells, etc.).

- Highly sensitive introverts are more emotionally reactive and experience negativity more intensely.

- Highly sensitive introverts are more empathic and can suffer more over the negative feelings of others.

Armed with this awareness, you can see how important it is to be your own best advocate—to reclaim some of your time, energy, and decision-making power so you can be as physically, mentally, and emotionally healthy as you desire to be.

Put any guilt or hesitancy aside, knowing that taking care of yourself means that you are also doing your best for your family, friends, and work associates. Self-care is a good thing. Put on your own oxygen mask first before helping others, right?

On a final note, as a fellow introvert, I'd like to thank you for reading this book and supporting my work in supporting introverts. My goal always is to provide proven, practical, and actionable strategies for living a better life. I hope I've achieved that for you.

Resource List

Introduction

Quiet: The Power of Introverts in a World That Can't Stop Talking, Susan Cain

TED Talk, The Power of Introverts, Susan Cain

Psychological Types, Carl Jung

Quiet Influence: The Introvert's Guide to Making a Difference, Jennifer B. Kahnweiler

Chapter 2: Practice Mindful Fitness

T'ai Chi Ch'uan for Health and Self-Defense: Philosophy and Practice, T. T. Liang

ChiRunning: A Revolutionary Approach to Effortless, Injury-Free Running, Danny Dreyer

Chapter 4: Get Plenty of Sleep

Sleep Soundly Every Night, Feel Fantastic Every Day: A Doctor's Guide to Solving Your Sleep Problems, Robert Rosenberg

Chapter 7: Body and Skin Care Rituals

Daily Rituals: How Artists Work, Mason Currey

Chapter 8: Creating Your Introvert Retreat

10-Minute Declutter: The Stress-Free Habit for Simplifying Your Home, S.J. Scott and Barrie Davenport

The Life-Changing Magic of Tidying Up: The Japanese Art of Decluttering and Organizing, Marie Kondo

Chapter 9: Practice Mindfulness

Peace of Mindfulness: Everyday Rituals to Conquer Anxiety and Claim Unlimited Inner Peace, Barrie Davenport

10-Minute Mindfulness: 71 Habits for Living in the Present Moment, S.J. Scott and Barrie Davenport

Guided Mindfulness Meditation Series 1: A Complete Guided Mindfulness Meditation Program from Jon Kabat-Zinn, Jon Kabat-Zinn

Chapter 12: Explore Creative Outlets

The Artist's Way: A Spiritual Path to Higher Creativity, Julia Cameron

Chapter 14: Enforce Digital Breaks

The Power of Off: The Mindful Way to Stay Sane in a Virtual World, Nancy Colier

Chapter 15: Treat Mental Health Problems

Feeling Good: The New Mood Therapy, David D. Burns

Cognitive Behavioral Therapy Made Simple: 10 Strategies for Managing Anxiety,

Depression, Anger, Panic, and Worry, Seth J. Gillihan

Chapter 16: Find Vitality and Meaning

The Untethered Soul: The Journey beyond Yourself, Michael A. Singer

Path to Passion course, Barrie Davenport

The Passion Journal: 102 Powerful Prompts to Crush Self-Doubt and Unlock a Remarkable Life, Barrie Davenport

Declutter Your Mind: How to Stop Worrying, Relieve Anxiety, and Eliminate Negative Thinking, S.J. Scott and Barrie Davenport

The Power of Now: A Guide to Spiritual Enlightenment, Eckhart Tolle

Loving What Is: Four Questions That Can Change Your Life, Byron Katie

Flow: The Psychology of Optimal Experience, Mihaly Csikszentmihalyi

Mindset: The New Psychology of Success, Carol Dweck

Man's Search for Meaning, Viktor E. Frankl

Emotional Intelligence 2.0, Travis Bradberry and Jean Greaves

Emotional Intelligence: A 21-Day Step by Step Guide to Mastering Social Skills, Improve Your Relationships, and Boost Your EQ, David Clark

Chapter 17: Create Emotional Outlets and Buffers

Finely-Tuned: How to Thrive as a Highly Sensitive Person or Empath, Barrie Davenport

The Highly Sensitive Person: How to Thrive When the World Overwhelms You, Elaine N. Aron

The Mindfulness Journal: Daily Practices, Writing Prompts, and Reflections for Living in The Present Moment, Barrie Davenport and S.J. Scott

How to Be an Imperfectionist: The New Way to Self-Acceptance, Fearless Living, and Freedom from Perfectionism, Stephen Guise

Radical Acceptance: Embracing Your Life with the Heart of a Buddha, Tara Brach

The Gifts of Imperfection: Let Go of Who You Think You're Supposed to Be and Embrace Who You Are, Brené Brown

References

Introduction

TED Talk, The Power of Introverts, Susan Cain, https://www.ted.com/talks/susan_cain_the_power_of_introverts

Myers-Briggs Type Indicator, https://www.myersbriggs.org/my-mbti-personality-type/mbti-basics/home.htm?bhcp=1

Quiet Revolution Personality Test, https://www.quietrev.com/the-introvert-test/

Quiet Influence: The Introvert's Guide to Making a Difference, Jennifer B. Kahnweiler, https://www.rd.com/health/wellness/introvert-personality-strengths/

Thoughts from Places: The Tour, John Green, https://www.goodreads.com/quotes/1050856-writing-is-something-you-do-alone-it-s-a-profession-for

Winifred Gallagher, https://www.cnn.com/2012/03/18/opinion/cain-introverts-power/index.html

Section 1: Physical Self-Care

"Study Sheds New Light on Relationship between Personality and Health" (2014), https://www.nottingham.ac.uk/news/pressreleases/2014/december/study-sheds-new-light-on-relationship-between-personality-and-health.aspx

"Personality Plays Role in Body Weight, According to Study" (2011). http://www.apa.org/news/press/releases/2011/07/personality-weight.aspx

Chapter 2: Practice Mindful Fitness

DoYogaWithMe, https://www.doyogawithme.com/

Online Tai Chi Lessons, https://www.onlinetaichilessons.com/

T'ai chi For Life, http://www.taichi-exercises.com/tai-chi-for-life-app/

Learn Qigong Online, http://www.learnqigongonline.com/

Zi Gong Meditation Relaxation, https://play.google.com/store/apps/details?id=com.excelatlife.motivation&hl=en

Ballet for Adult Beginners, https://www.danceclass.com/ballet-for-adult-beginners.html

"Rebounding: The Small Trampoline Exercise That's Addictively Fun," https://liveboldandbloom.com/02/health/rebounding-the-small-trampoline-exercise-thats-addictively-fun

Chapter 4: Get Plenty of Sleep

Best Mattress Brand, "Pillow Personalities," https://www.bestmattress-brand.org/pillow-personalities/

"Nightmares Affect the Experience of Sleep Quality but Not Sleep Architecture: An Ambulatory Polysomnographic Study," https://www.ncbi.nlm.nih.gov/pmc/articles/PMC4579510/

Calm, www.calm.com

Headspace, https://www.headspace.com/

Chapter 5: Pay Attention to Your Body

"Mind-Body Research Moves towards the Mainstream," https://www.ncbi.nlm.nih.gov/pmc/articles/PMC1456909/

"Massage Therapy for Health Purposes," https://nccih.nih.gov/health/massage/massageintroduction.htm

"What Are the Risks of Sitting Too Much?" https://www.mayoclinic.org/healthy-lifestyle/adult-health/expert-answers/sitting/faq-20058005

"Health Experts Have Figured Out How Much Time You Should Sit Each Day," https://www.washingtonpost.com/news/wonk/wp/2015/06/02/medical-researchers-have-figured-out-how-much-time-is-okay-to-spend-sitting-each-day/?noredirect=on&utm_term=.0620799826fc

"[Ikea Hack] My Standing Desk / Treadmill Desk—Part 2," http://melissadinwiddie.com/ikea-hack-standing-desk-treadmill-desk-part-2/

"Mild Dehydration Impairs Cognitive Performance and Mood of Men," https://www.cambridge.org/core/journals/british-journal-of-nutrition/article/mild-dehydration-impairs-cognitive-performance-and-mood-of-men/3388AB36B8DF73E844C9AD19271A75BF

"Even Mild Dehydration Can Alter Mood," https://today.uconn.edu/2012/02/even-mild-dehydration-can-alter-mood/

Chapter 6: The Introvert Diet

"High Glycemic Index Diet as a Risk Factor for Depression: Analyses from the Women's Health Initiative," https://academic.oup.com/ajcn/article/102/2/454/4564524

"Fast-Food and Commercial Baked Goods Consumption and the Risk of Depression," https://www.ncbi.nlm.nih.gov/pubmed/21835082

"Fermented Foods, Neuroticism, and Social Anxiety: An Interaction Model," https://www.ncbi.nlm.nih.gov/pubmed/25998000

"The Effects of Probiotics on Depressive Symptoms in Humans: A Systematic Review," https://www.ncbi.nlm.nih.gov/pmc/articles/PMC5319175/

"Omega-3 Supplementation Lowers Inflammation and Anxiety in Medical Students: A Randomized Controlled Trial," https://www.ncbi.nlm.nih.gov/pubmed/21784145

"Omega-3 Fatty Acids and Depression: Scientific Evidence and Biological Mechanisms," https://www.ncbi.nlm.nih.gov/pmc/articles/PMC3976923/

"Rapid Recovery from Major Depression Using Magnesium Treatment," http://www.george-eby-research.com/html/magnesium-for-depression.pdf

"Magnesium for Treatment-Resistant Depression: A Review and Hypothesis," https://www.ncbi.nlm.nih.gov/pubmed/19944540

"Vitamin B6 (Pyridoxine)," http://pennstatehershey.adam. com/content.aspx?productId=107&pid=33&gid=000337

"The Effect of Methylated Vitamin B Complex on Depressive and Anxiety Symptoms and Quality of Life in Adults with Depression," https://www.ncbi.nlm.nih.gov/pubmed/23738221

Chapter 7: Body and Skin Care Rituals

"A Hot Bath Has Benefits Similar to Exercise," https://theconversation. com/a-hot-bath-has-benefits-similar-to-exercise-74600

"Make Your Own Restorative Eucalyptus Mint Bath Oil," https://www.onegoodthingbyjillee.com/2015/05/make-your-own-restorative-eucalyptus-mint-bath-oil.html

"Four Essential Oils to Help You Beat Depression," https://liveboldandbloom.com/08/product-reviews/essential-oils-for-anxiety

Chapter 8: Creating Your Introvert Retreat

"Interactions of Top-Down and Bottom-Up Mechanisms in Human Visual Cortex," https://www.ncbi.nlm.nih.gov/pubmed/21228167

"Living with Less. A Lot Less," https://www.nytimes. com/2013/03/10/opinion/sunday/living-with-less-a-lot-less. html?pagewanted=2&_r=0&hp

"Five Cool Prefab Backyard Sheds You Can Buy Right Now," https://www.curbed.com/2018/3/9/17091786/prefab-house-shed-for-sale-buy-backyard-office-studio

"Thirty-Seven Smart DIY Hanging Bed Tutorials and Ideas to Do,"https://homesthetics.net/diy-hanging-bed/

"APA Gains Sanity: Introverts Not Nuts," https://www.psychologytoday.com/us/ blog/self-promotion-introverts/201206/ apa-gains-sanity-introverts-not-nuts

"Revenge of the Introvert," https://www.psychologytoday.com/ us/articles/201009/revenge-the-introvert

"Relationship of Myers Briggs Type Indicator Personality Characteristics to Suicidality in Affective Disorder Patients," https://www.sciencedirect.com/science/article/pii/ S0022395601000437

Chapter 9: Practice Mindfulness

"Mindfulness Practice: Eight Powerful Benefits," https:// liveboldandbloom.com/02/mindfulness/mindfulness-practice

Chapter 10: Spend Time in Nature

"The National Human Activity Pattern Survey (NHAPS): A Resource for Assessing Exposure to Environmental Pollutants," https://www.nature.com/articles/7500165

"Eleven Scientific Reasons You Should Be Spending More Time Outside," http://www.businessinsider.com/scientific-benefits-of-nature-outdoors-2016-4/#1-improved-short-term-memory-1

"Circadian Entrainment to the Natural Light-Dark Cycle across Seasons and the Weekend," https://www.cell.com/ current-biology/fulltext/S0960-9822(16)31522-6

"The Struggles of an Introverted Adventurer,"
https://www.adventure-journal.com/2018/03/
the-struggles-of-an-introverted-adventurer/

Chapter 11: Read for Pleasure

"Why Readers, Scientifically, Are the Best People to Fall in Love With," https://www.elitedaily.com/life/culture/date-reader-readers-best-people-fall-love-scientifically-proven/662017

Bookclubz, https://bookclubz.com/

Book Club Meetups, https://www.meetup.com/topics/bookclub/?_cookie-check=ESFGOcJzxk453xL5

My-bookclub.com, https://www.my-bookclub.com/

The Rumpus Book Club, http://therumpus.net/bookclub/

"Is Listening to a Book 'Cheating?'" https://www.washingtonpost.com/news/answer-sheet/wp/2016/07/31/is-listening-to-a-book-a-cheating/?noredirect=on&utm_term=.d49cfa0761f9

Chapter 12: Explore Creative Outlets

"Sixteen Super Successful Introverts," https://www.huffingtonpost.com/2015/08/15/famous-introverts_n_3733400.html

"How BIS/BAS and Psycho-Behavioral Variables Distinguish between Social Withdrawal Subtypes during Emerging Adulthood," https://www.sciencedirect.com/science/article/pii/S0191886917304920

"Why Introverts Need 'Creative Space,'" https://introvertdear.com/news/introverts-need-creative-space/

"Reduction of Cortisol Levels and Participants' Responses Following Art Making," https://www.tandfonline.com/doi/abs/10.1080/07421656.2016.1166832?journalCode=uart20&#.V2GKm-YrI6g

Chapter 14: Enforce Digital Breaks

"The World UNPLUGGED," https://theworldunplugged.wordpress.com/

"How Smartphone Addiction Is Affecting Our Physical and Mental Health," https://www.seattletimes.com/life/wellness/how-smartphone-addiction-is-affecting-our-physical-and-mental-health/

"Exposure to Room Light before Bedtime Suppresses Melatonin Onset and Shortens Melatonin Duration in Humans," https://www.ncbi.nlm.nih.gov/pmc/articles/PMC3047226/, https://academic.oup.com/jcem/article/96/3/E463/2597236

"Annual Sleep in America Poll Exploring Connections with Communications Technology Use and Sleep," https://sleepfoundation.org/media-center/press-release/annual-sleep-america-poll-exploring-connections-communications-technology-use-

"How Modern Life Affects Our Physical and Mental Health," https://www.medicalnewstoday.com/articles/318230.php

Chapter 15: Treat Mental Health Problems

"What Are Anxiety Disorders?" https://www.webmd.com/anxiety-panic/guide/anxiety-disorders#1

"Symptoms of Depression," https://www.webmd.com/depression/guide/detecting-depression#1

"Adding Psychotherapy to Antidepressant Medication in Depression and Anxiety Disorders: A Meta-Analysis," https://www.ncbi.nlm.nih.gov/pmc/articles/PMC3918025/

"Using CBT Effectively for Treating Depression and Anxiety," https://www.mdedge.com/psychiatry/article/82695/anxiety-disorders/using-cbt-effectively-treating-depression-and-anxiety

"Public Attitudes about Mental Health," https://ropercenter.cornell.edu/public-attitudes-mental-health/

Chapter 16: Find Vitality and Meaning

Path to Passion, https://liveboldandbloom.com/path-passion-sp

"How to Find Your Passion and Do the Work You Love," https://liveboldandbloom.com/03/passion-in-life/how-to-find-passion

"Emotional Plasticity: Conditions and Effects of Improving Emotional Competence in Adulthood," https://www.ncbi.nlm.nih.gov/pubmed/21443316

"Emotional Intelligence Test," https://bit.ly/2IExHRS

"How to Improve Emotional Intelligence: 10 Tips for Increasing Self-Awareness," https://www.6seconds.org/2018/02/27/emotional-intelligence-tips-awareness/

"Introverts, Being Spiritual Doesn't Have to Be Loud," https://introvertdear.com/news/how-to-find-peace-as-a-spiritual-introvert/

Chapter 17: Create Emotional Outlets and Buffers

"Are You Highly Sensitive?" https://hsperson.com/test/highly-sensitive-test/

"Pets Provide 'Unique' Support to People with Mental Illness," https://www.medicalnewstoday.com/articles/314668.php

"Personality Differences between Dog and Cat Owners," https://www.psychologytoday.com/us/blog/canine-corner/201002/personality-differences-between-dog-and-cat-owners

"What Dog Breed Should You Get Based on Your Personality Type?" https://www.purewow.com/entertainment/What-Dog-Breed-Should-You-Get-Based-on-Your-Personality-Type

Conclusion

"What We Have Learned about Gifted Children," http://www.gifteddevelopment.com/articles/what-we-have-learned-about-gifted-children

Did You Like *Self-Care for Introverts*?

Thank you so much for purchasing *Self-Care for Introverts: 17 Soothing Rituals for Peace in a Hectic World.* I'm honored by the trust you've placed in me and my work by choosing this book to better understand introverts and how to improve your life. I truly hope you've enjoyed it and found it useful for your life.

I'd like to ask you for a small favor. Would you please take just a minute to leave a review for this book on Amazon? This feedback will help me continue to write the kind of books that will best serve you. If you really loved the book, please let me know!

Other Books and Journals You Might Enjoy from Barrie Davenport

- *201 Relationship Questions Journal: A Diary for Two to Build Trust and Emotional Intimacy*
- *The Life Passion Journal: 102 Powerful Prompts to Crush Self-Doubt and Unlock a Remarkable Life*
- *The Mindfulness Journal: Daily Practices, Writing Prompts, and Reflections for Living in the Present Moment*
- *Mindful Relationship Habits: 25 Practices for Couples to Enhance Intimacy, Nurture Closeness, and Grow a Deeper Connection*
- *201 Relationship Questions: The Couple's Guide to Building Trust and Emotional Intimacy*
- *Emotional Abuse Breakthrough: How to Speak Up, Set Boundaries, and Break the Cycle of Manipulation and Control with Your Abusive Partner*
- *Emotional Abuse Breakthrough Scripts: 107 Empowering Responses and Boundaries to Use with Your Abuser*
- *Signs of Emotional Abuse: How to Recognize the Patterns of Narcissism, Manipulation, and Control in Your Love Relationship*
- *Building Confidence: Get Motivated, Overcome Social Fear, Be Assertive, and Empower Your Life for Success*

- *Peace of Mindfulness: Everyday Rituals to Conquer Anxiety and Claim Unlimited Inner Peace*

- *Finely-Tuned: How to Thrive as a Highly Sensitive Person or Empath*

- *Self-Discovery Questions: 155 Breakthrough Questions to Accelerate Massive Action*

- *Confidence Hacks: 99 Small Actions to Massively Boost Your Confidence*

- *10-Minute Declutter: The Stress-Free Habit for Simplifying Your Home*

- *10-Minute Digital Declutter: The Simple Habit to Eliminate Technology Overload*

- *10-Minute Mindfulness: 71 Habits for Living in the Present Moment*

- *Declutter Your Mind: How to Stop Worrying, Relieve Anxiety, and Eliminate Negative Thinking*

- *Sticky Habits: How to Achieve Your Goals without Quitting and Create Unbreakable Habits Starting with Five Minutes a Day*

- *The 52-Week Life Passion Project: Uncover Your Life Passion*